The Diabetic's Total Health and Happiness Book

REVISED AND EXPANDED

The Diabetic's Total Health and Happiness Book

4TH EDITION

June Biermann

Barbara Toohey

JEREMY P. TARCHER/PENGUIN
a member of Penguin Group (USA) Inc.
New York

Every effort has been made to ensure that the information contained in this book is complete and accurate. However, neither the publisher nor the authors are engaged in rendering professional advice or services to the individual reader. The ideas, procedures, and suggestions contained in this book are not intended as a substitute for consulting with your physician. All matters regarding your health require medical supervision. Neither the authors nor the publisher shall be liable or responsible for any loss or damage allegedly arising from any information or suggestion in this book.

While the authors have made every effort to provide accurate telephone numbers and Internet addresses at the time of publication, neither the publisher nor the authors assume any responsibility for errors, or for changes that occur after publication.

Most Tarcher/Penguin books are available at special quantity discounts for bulk purchase for sales promotions, premiums, fund-raising, and educational needs. Special books or book excerpts also can be created to fit specific needs. For details, write Penguin Group (USA) Inc. Special Markets, 375 Hudson Street, New York, NY 10014.

Jeremy P. Tarcher/Penguin
a member of
Penguin Group (USA) Inc.
375 Hudson Street
New York, NY 10014
www.penguin.com

Library of Congress Cataloging-in-Publication Data

Biermann, June.
    The diabetic's total health and happiness book / June Biermann and Barbara Toohey.—
4th ed.
        p. cm.
    Previous editions published under title: The diabetic's total health book.
    ISBN 1-58542-230-4
        1. Diabetes—Popular works.   2. Diabetes—Diet therapy—Recipes.   3. Diabetes—
Miscellanea.   I. Toohey, Barbara.   II. Biermann, June. Diabetic's total health book.
III. Title.
RC660.4.B54   2003   2003044778
616.4'62—dc21

Printed in the United States of America
1   3   5   7   9   10   8   6   4   2

Book design by Tanya Maiboroda

In memory of Betty Annis
for years and years and years of
total love, encouragement, and support

Contents

Foreword

"Our remedies oft in ourselves do lie."

—SHAKESPEARE, *ALL'S WELL THAT ENDS WELL*, I, i, 231

This is a lovely book. It expresses a "can do" attitude. We learn why people with diabetes should actively participate in their own medical care. The authors remind us of how well a diabetic person feels when the diabetes stays controlled. We come to understand that no obstacle is totally insurmountable. Prudent eating habits, sports and exercise, and a positive mental outlook, as well as more innovative techniques like laughter and hug therapy, become integral parts of total health.

Fostering these active-positive attitudes adds to the quality of life whether or not one has diabetes. Stress lessens and optimism flowers. Good self-care is accentuated.

This book discusses many agreeable activities, and yet the authors suggest that not every activity, no matter how beneficial it may seem, is necessarily the proper choice for every individual. They wisely point out the possible options so that we can make personal choices.

Savor this book; it is vintage Biermann-Toohey. They have used diabetes as a role model for coping with life. They have shown us how simple living and thinking will embellish a lifestyle. Since they themselves are complete people, we should consider their views and find ways to incorporate those thoughts and activities that we find personally compatible. Here is a book that makes us think. Surely, this is the mark of something new that is worthwhile.

FRED WHITEHOUSE, M.D.
Chief, Division of Endocrinology and Metabolism
Henry Ford Hospital
Detroit, Michigan
Past President, American Diabetes Association

Changes: For Worse and for Better

In the ten years since the last edition of *The Diabetic's Total Health Book,* diabetes has been on a rampage, having increased by a whopping 33 percent. Type 2 (noninsulin-dependent) statistics are even more distressing. It has increased by 70 percent in the thirty to thirty-nine age group. In those aged forty to forty-nine, it's up by 40 percent and among those over fifty it's now 31 percent more prevalent than before. Now more and more children and young people are developing type 2—known in the trade as MODY (Maturity Onset Diabetes in the Young).

All this totals out at approximately 800,000 new cases of diabetes a year. And that figure is undoubtedly low since so many cases remain undiagnosed.

In order to prevent or at least forestall the burgeoning development of diabetes, U.S. health officials are urging all overweight Americans forty-five or older to be regularly screened for a condition they now call "pre-diabetes." (Formerly it was known as "glucose intolerance.") It is estimated that 16 million Americans between the ages of forty and seventy-four have this condition. Two blood-sugar indicators of "pre-diabetes" are a measurement between 140 and 199 and an overnight fasting measurement of between 110 and 125.

If pre-diabetes is diagnosed, studies indicate that by making simple diet changes, losing weight, and embarking on a moderate exercise program, the number of those going on to full-blown diabetes can be reduced by about 60 percent.

American eating habits and the resulting weight gain are in part responsible for the increase in diabetes. We can also point an accusatory finger at stress and the decrease in exercise.

For this reason, we felt that the time had come to start pounding the tom-toms even harder, delivering the word on new ways to prevent, delay, and control diabetes. As in our previous editions, we want to continue focusing positively on your health rather than negatively on your disease, taking the holistic approach of considering the total mind, body, and spirit of you. But as you see from the new title, *The Diabetic's Total Health and **Happiness** Book,* we've added another equally important goal.

THE PURSUIT OF HAPPINESS

People with diabetes, as we've learned from experience, are particularly susceptible to another and even more insidious disease. This condition was described by Susan R. Michael, R.N., CDE, at an American Association of Diabetes Educators Conference. She named it "Chronic Sorrow." It is a stage of mourning—feeling depressed or sorrowful—that can occur throughout your entire life as a diabetic. Although you are at particular risk for chronic sorrow at the time of diagnosis, even after you think you've got it cured, it keeps coming back like a song—or more like a dirge. It can sometimes grow and grow to the point that you develop what attorneys who are trying to jack up the settlements in personal injury cases call "hedonic loss." This means the loss of the ability to experience pleasure and enjoy life. The specter of diabetes is always looming, blocking out the sunshine.

We think it's time to let the sunshine back into your life, to recognize the fact that your happiness is just as important as your health. In fact, they go together like a horse and carriage. You're very unlikely to have one without the other. We want this book to help you attain both in full measure.

BOOK SURFING WITH DIABETILINKS

We recently spent a year as "content providers" (computerese for writers) on a diabetes website. It was an enlightening period in more ways than one. We found it particularly fascinating to see how people in the modern world skip around a site, following up links to information that interests them, then returning to the home-page base to seek out and follow up on other links. We liked the possibilities of this way of communication and so we've incorporated it in this edition with DiabetiLinks.

You will have the basic book (corresponding to the home page) and from time to time as you read along there will be a DiabetiLink to pages in the back of the book, where you'll find embellishments on the topic you've been reading about or related subjects or material directed specifically to type 1 (insulin-dependent) or type 2, etc. Here's where you'll also find the contrarian position—an opposite opinion on the topic discussed in the body of the book. If you follow up on these DiabetiLinks at the end of each entry you will find the page number, to get back to where you were in the basic book. You can go read each DiabetiLink as you come to it, or pick and choose among the links, or ignore them entirely, marching resolutely through the book, waiting to read all the links when you've finished the basic book. It's Freedom Hall here. Read what you will when you will as you will. We just hope that eventually you will read everything and file it all in your mental archives for ready access.

Now let's boot up and log on.

The Gift of Diabetes

· · · · · · · · · · · · · · · ·

In 1999, Roberto Benigni's film *Life Is Beautiful* won three Academy Awards. You may remember him eagerly clambering over the backs of chairs to reach the stage. In his acceptance speech for Best Actor, Benigni thanked his parents, "who gave me the greatest gift: poverty." Not that being poor was more fun than a barrel of monkeys for a young boy in rural Italy, but overcoming this poverty with humor and intelligence and dedication brought him to his acting, writing, and directing career and ultimately to the Academy triumph.

Although you will surely doubt it now, someday you may be thankful for the "gift of diabetes." Just like poverty, diabetes is no barrel of monkeys, and you certainly would rather not have it. But if you overcome your diabetes with humor and intelligence and dedication, you will come to realize that truly life is beautiful—not just in spite of diabetes, but, strangely enough, sometimes *because* of it.

HEALTH THROUGH THE GIFT OF DIABETES

There's an old saying that, like most old sayings, contains a lot of truth: "The secret of a long life is to have a chronic disease and take good care of it." This is even more applicable to diabetes than to other chronic diseases. We call diabetes "the more-so disease." Aside from the blood-sugar testing and the medications you may need to take, everything you should do for your diabetes is just what everyone should do for their general health—only more so. As you'll read in this book, exercising, keeping weight down, not smoking, taking flu shots, eating healthy foods, not overindulging in alcohol, getting enough sleep, and the myriad other good health habits that everyone should acquire are what you should do to take care of your diabetes.

But since these health habits are an integral part of your diabetes therapy and you have the diabetes sword of Damocles suspended over your head threatening to drop and lop off some part of your anatomy that you would prefer to keep intact, you're much less likely to ignore the good health practices than a nondiabetic would. Example: Nondiabetic Barbara tries to follow the diabetic ways of good health. And for the most part she does. But although she perpetually would like to lose around ten pounds, they tend to stay with her. Why? Because if something appears on the table that she would really like to have, she frequently indulges herself "just this once." June, on the other hand, virtually never indulges in this way. She knows it will show up on her blood-sugar monitor readings and she also knows that if those readings are perpetually high, she may be on the road to ketoacidosis, a condition that signals that your body is burning your fat, and *that* road could lead to diabetic coma and . . . well, you get the picture. Diabetes is a great motivator to do the right thing.

As Kathy, a young diabetic woman, said in a letter to us, "When I'm at dinner and there's a big luscious piece of chocolate cake there before me, although I really love chocolate, I stop and think. I think about my feet that I really like to walk on and my eyes that I really like to see out of and my kidneys that I really want to keep doing whatever it is they do. Then I have no trouble taking a very tiny bite and leaving all the rest."

DISEASE AND HEALTH

We once heard a doctor make an interesting distinction between disease and health. He said you can be completely free from disease and yet be unhealthy: rundown, flabby, sallow, sluggish, unproductive, depressed—or, in other words, a physical, mental, and emotional mess. On the other hand, you can have a definite chronic illness like diabetes and yet be healthy—strong, lithe, lean, vigorous, alert, productive, and enthusiastic; or, in other words, a physical, mental, and emotional triumph. (Think of cancer victim—and survivor!—cycling champion Lance Armstrong, four-time winner of the Tour de France.)

We want to help you achieve your own kind of triumph by helping you change your outlook. Although diabetes may be a motivating force to keep you on the straight and narrow rather than the crooked and wide, you should think of yourself as making positive changes in your lifestyle not because you have diabetes, but because you want to be a healthy, happy, productive person. The changes we're recommending are not restrictive; they are expansive. They are the kinds of changes that every person who wants to enjoy life to the fullest should be making. But, alas, without the Gift of Diabetes, many of them just don't get around to it.

HAPPINESS THROUGH THE GIFT OF DIABETES

One lesson diabetes teaches you early on is that you're mortal. When that realization first hits you, at the time of your diagnosis, it's a terrible shock, especially if you've been just bouncing through life as oblivious as a puppy to the fact that you don't have all the time in the world to squander.

Of course, you could just give up and dwell in the shadow of the valley of death for the rest of your life and thereby blight your whole existence and that of your family and friends. But strangely enough, that's not the way it usually works. Author, lecturer, and guru of love Leo F. Buscaglia said that the happiest people he knew were those with a sense of their own mortality. They realize that they have a limited number of days and that each one is precious and should be enjoyed to the fullest. He exemplified this in his own life. In his later years he developed a chronic heart condition, and he knew that any day could be his last. Did he sit around coddling himself and mourning his fate? Not on your life—or his! He packed every day with joyful experiences for himself and all those around him. The year before he died he traveled throughout the United States, Europe, and Asia.

The evening of the night he died he had a celebratory dinner with friends, enjoying to the fullest the good food, good wine, and good companionship. The morning after his death this note was found on his typewriter: "Every moment lost in unhappiness is a moment of happiness lost. Don't lose a moment!" Leo didn't. It's significant that his middle initial, F, stood for Felice, the Italian word for happy.

Recently, a very close friend suffered such a severe stroke that everyone—especially the doctors—thought she was a goner. But she rose from the ashes and even though she's now spending most of her time either in a wheelchair or undergoing enervating physical and occupational therapy, she is chipper as a cricket, never depressed or complaining about her lot in life. When friends remark on this, she always says, "I'm lucky just to be alive. I'm determined to enjoy every minute I have."

So thanks to the Gift of Diabetes, you now know how precious your life is and how much joy is out there just for the taking. Only a fool would not grab it with both hands.

WHY DOES HAPPINESS BREED GOOD HEALTH?

Science hasn't done a very good job at figuring out why happiness is so healthy and at explaining what's going on in the body when it's enjoying itself and wallowing in happy feelings. Does it have something to do with those endorphins that exercise produces giving that famous "runner's high"? Probably not. Endorphins really have less to do with joy than with easing the perception of pain. One fairly new theory is that oxytocin, a hormone secreted by the pituitary, might have something to do with feelings of satisfaction and euphoria, but so far most of the experiments have been limited to laboratory rats— you know those lucky guys who are always getting their diabetes cured. (Maybe *that's* what makes them so happy rather than the oxytocin.)

It's true that there hasn't been much human research done on happiness. As Dr. Redford B. Williams of Duke University Medical Center says, "Our focus is always on what's making people sick so we can fix it." They concentrate on observing happiness from a negative perspective, that is to say, "happiness is healthy because it spares us the negative impacts of anxiety and depression." Dr. Williams says the problem is that it's hard to replicate happiness in a laboratory. "If we could come up with an easy experimental manipulation to make subjects happy, we wouldn't be sitting around here studying anger and depression all the time."

But there are some positive souls studying happiness from the upside. Robert Ornstein, Ph.D., and David Sobel, M.D., authors of *Healthy Pleasures,* say that experiencing pleasure "pays off not only in immediate enjoyment but also in better health." They take the somewhat radical position that people are increasingly viewing themselves as fragile and vulnerable, ready to develop cancer, heart disease, or something else at the slightest provocation. In the name of health they give up many of life's enjoyments. Their point is that worrying too much about anything—be it calories, salt, sugar, cancer, or cholesterol—is bad for you and that living optimistically with pleasure, zest, and commitment is good. And, we might add, good for your health and for your diabetes.

≫**DiabetiLink #1:** New Study of Happy People (See p. 259)

Let us now unwrap the Gift of Diabetes and see what good things are waiting there for you.

PART 1

A STRONG BODY

What makes for good physical health? Heredity, of course is a major factor, but it's a little late to select new ancestors if yours have left you with a few holes in your genes, such as your tendency toward diabetes. What counts now is what you do with what you've got: the food and the chemicals you do or don't put into your body and the activities you do or don't ask your body to perform.

One surgeon general's report on health promotion and disease prevention laid it on the line, stating that "as many as half of American deaths are attributed to unhealthy behavior or lifestyle." To express these concepts in automotive terms, at birth you may have been given a Rolls-Royce or a VW Beetle. That you can't change. But you are the one who is responsible for filling with fuel and driving and maintaining the machine you were born with. Whether you have a long lifetime of efficient, carefree transportation from your body or a quick, sputtering trip to the junkyard is up to you.

CHAPTER 1

Self-Control

. . . .

Although in this book we're emphasizing your health rather than your disease, it's a given that if you're going to pursue optimum health and maximum happiness, you're going to have to start from a base of good diabetes control. If your diabetes is out of control, it's a wretched stress on the body, it opens the door for all kinds of minor and major infections, and it just plain makes you feel rotten—exhausted, listless, and sometimes even nauseated. But that's not the worst part. If you know anything about diabetes, you know that long-term, out-of-control blood sugar is what causes the dread complications you always hear about and keep trying to push out of your mind. But they won't be pushed out. The worry is always there when your blood sugars are consistently running high or are bouncing all over the map. But this is one worry you can get rid of with good control, because—now hear this—the majority of the leading experts in the field of diabetes now concur that *keeping blood sugar in the normal range will prevent complications.* The 1993 release of the results of Diabetes Control and Complications Trial (DCCT) proved that for type 1's. The next major test will undoubtedly prove the same for type 2's. In fact, one already has: the Kumamoto study in Japan tracked 110 type 2's and not only did they have the same improvement in eye and kidney disease as the type 1's in the DCCT, but there also was a 50 percent reduction in cardiac events.

That good control, that magic of normal blood sugar, is up to you. Fortunately, the tools of good control are now available to you. (If you had to go and get diabetes, at least you picked the right time.)

If you've been regularly testing your blood sugar for quite a while, you know how to do it, you know its importance, and you don't need us to give you a hype and hard sell on the topic, you may want to skip the next few paragraphs. But you should check out this link for important information.

➤ **DiabetiLink #2:** For Veteran Blood-Sugar Testers (See p. 260)

BLOOD-SUGAR TESTING

Testing your blood sugar or, in health professional language, self-monitoring of blood glucose (SMBG), has been described as the most important advance in the management of diabetes since the discovery of insulin in the 1920s. Although that may be something of an exaggeration, it's hard to overstate the importance of doing your own blood-sugar testing. After all, our diabetes is all about blood-sugar (glucose) levels. When levels are too low or too high, we face the consequences. Hypoglycemia (low blood sugar) can lead to dizziness, unconsciousness, or even (rarely) death. Hyperglycemia (high blood sugar) over the long term can lead to serious complications.

The Good News

When June was diagnosed back in the Dark Ages of Diabetes, she could check her blood-glucose level only by visiting a clinical laboratory. Now you can check your own blood-sugar level in a minute or less at home, or just about anywhere else you might happen to be. Testing is easy, convenient, and highly reliable thanks to the development of small, battery-powered glucose meters that determine glucose levels when a small drop of blood is put on a disposable test strip. The meters are inexpensive and getting less so every day. Sometimes, with rebates and trade-ins, they're even free.

The Bad News

As the price of meters keeps coming down, the price of strips doesn't. It's the old razor/razor blade system. They sell you the razor for very little and make their money on the blades. Strips now run from 52 to 80 cents each. You can pay even more if you use certain pharmacies or if the supplier has to bill your health insurance. It's easy to see that the price of test strips adds up to a not-so-pretty penny for frequent testers.

Incidentally, almost all insurance companies, realizing that good control keeps you out of the hospital and ultimately saves them money, are at least partially paying for meters and strips. Even Medicare now pays a major portion of the cost of meters and strips for both type 1's (insulin-taking) and type 2's (non-insulin-taking).

Another new development is that as the prices of strips ascend, it is an incentive for some astute entrepreneurs to develop less expensive, what you might call "generic," strips for the most popular meters.

Who Should Test?

We emphatically believe that everyone with diabetes should test for blood sugar. Very young or very frail or enfeebled persons may need help in testing, but everyone should test regularly and learn how to take action when the blood sugar is too high or low. With the guidance of a physician or diabetes educator, type 1's will need to know how to lower their blood sugar with small injections of fast-acting insulin and how to raise their blood sugar the fastest and most effective way with glucose tablets.

Type 2's will need to test and record their highs and lows (and the circumstances surrounding them) in order to make it possible for their health-care professionals to make adjustments in their medications and/or diet. Not all oral hypoglycemics (diabetes pills) will cause low blood sugars. *Diabetes Self-Management* reported that those that *can* are Glucatrol, DiaBeta, Glynase, Micronase, Amaryl, Star-lix, and Prandin. Those that do *not* are Glucophage and Avandia, either used singly or in combination.

How Frequently Should You Test?

It depends. Endocrinologist Dr. Steven V. Edelman (a card-carrying diabetic himself) is the founder of the Taking Control of Your Diabetes educational and motivational conferences. He points out that, "Some individuals who are elderly with *very* consistent daily schedules and whose diabetes is quite stable may only need to test once or twice a week. And more occasional but still regular testing may be suitable for a person with very well-controlled type 2 diabetes." Others need to test far more often. Dr. Edelman believes that "testing up to ten or fifteen times a day may be needed to achieve good control in persons on a multiple, daily, insulin-injection regimen or on an insulin pump, especially if they are very active and if they follow very different daily schedules for eating and exercising." But everyone is different. To find out how frequently and at what times you should test, talk to your physician or diabetes educator.

Be sure to ask them about those times when extra testing may be a good idea; for example:

- if you're sick
- if you think your blood sugar is low
- before you drive a car (or boat or motorcycle or snowmobile or even a motorized scooter!)
- before and after vigorous exercise
- when you make changes in your medication or diet
- when you are pregnant or considering becoming pregnant

What's Your Goal?

Again, it depends. The American Diabetes Association says that pre-meal glucose levels should be less than 115 milligrams daily, and after-meal glucose levels should be less than 140 milligrams. Blood glucose goals for people—especially the elderly and those with heart conditions—can often be higher than this. Talk to your doctor or diabetes educator to establish target blood-glucose levels that are right for you.

Why Bother to Test?

A diabetes educator friend of ours states simply, "You can't control what you don't monitor." Moreover, we think, you can't control if you *only* monitor. As strange as it may seem, lots of self-testers never do anything about their test results except admire the normal results and groan about the high ones! Dr. Edelman encourages his patients to get more actively involved in monitoring. "Don't just test and write the numbers down for your doctor or diabetes educator. Think about what that number means, why you are at that glucose level, and what you should do to correct the number. Think about how to avoid that problem again in the future." Sometimes you can figure out right away why a single glucose result was too high or too low. But much of the time it's a mystery. Fortunately, it's a mystery that you can usually solve. The solution is to keep track of your glucose levels, the medication you take, the food you eat, and your exercise. Your glucose logbook (or electronic logbook) will help you and your health-care team find patterns that cause the highs and the lows. Seeing progress can be very motivating, as it reminds you that you are gaining better control of your diabetes. And you will be learning that you are an individual and have your own distinctive case of diabetes.

CHOOSING YOUR GLUCOSE TEST SYSTEM

The first logical question to ask is, "What is the best meter?" There have been many studies of meter accuracy and reproducibility (meaning if you take several blood sugars one after another they will come out the same). Well then, based on these studies, what *is* the best meter? The cynic would answer that what turns out to be the best meter in the test is the one made by the company funding the test—and the cynic would probably be right. Would *you* spend a lot of money on a study that showed a rival meter had the edge on yours? Not likely.

But you needn't fret. All the meters on the market have to have FDA approval, so as a result there is much less risk of meter inaccuracy than of operator error—and *that* you have control over. There are lots of great test systems out there now—and more appearing every year. (Check the Resource Guide in each January issue of *Diabetes Forecast* for a list of the systems currently available and their features.) Be sure to talk to your pharmacist and other health-care team members for their opinions about the various brands. Diabetes nurse-educators are a particularly good source of this information because the representatives of the meter companies always beat a path to their doors the moment their "new and improved" meters come onto the market.

But ultimately your question should be not "What is the best meter?" but "What is the best meter for me?" You'll want to choose the test system that has the features most important to you. Speed? Portability? Amount of blood required? Ease of operation? Cost of strips? Ability to take blood for the test from the arm as well as the fingertips? (B. B. King's preference!) To be realistic, it often boils down to what your insurance or HMO is willing to provide for you. But above all, whatever meter you wind up with, be sure that someone, be it the person who sells the meter to you or your diabetes educator, gives you thorough instruction in its operation. It's that old devil operator error we mentioned. A misused meter giving you a wildly inaccurate reading is worse than no meter at all.

MONITORING OVERALL CONTROL

A dietitian who has had diabetes since she was a teenager was testing her pre-meal blood sugar at a restaurant and announced, "I'm at 183 (milligrams per deciliter). Does that mean I'm 183 going up, or 183 going down!" She makes a good point: any single blood-glucose test measures only a moment in time. While that's important so you can correct an immediate high or low blood sugar, what about the big picture, the long-range view of your blood-sugar control? Fortunately, now there are ways to find that out. By monitoring the amount of glucose that sticks to proteins in the blood it's possible to get an idea of what the average of continuous sugar levels has been over the preceding weeks or months. These "sticky proteins" are called glycated proteins. Here are the tests:

HbA1c: The best know glycated protein test is the glycated hemoglobin or glycohemoglobin test, commonly referred to as hemoglobin A1c (HbA1c). This test shows how your overall control has been over the past two to three months by analyzing how much glucose has bonded with the red blood cells. The ADA recommends that all persons with diabetes monitor their HbA1c levels at least twice per year. This test is usually performed in your doctor's office. Since the normal range varies with different laboratory tests, rather than asking what the numerical result of your test is you should ascertain the normal range for that particular laboratory and see where your test results fit on that scale. Your doctor can order the test from the laboratory, or you can buy one of the home test kits that lets you mail a fingerstick blood sample to a distant laboratory for analysis and return-mail notification. (Current prices range from $18.50 to $29.95.) These tests include:

Accu-Base Hemoglobin A1c Sample Collection Kit. Sold over-the-counter and includes postage-paid mailer. Results can be faxed, mailed, or e-mailed to the patient and/or the physician.

> Diabetes Technologies, Inc.
> P.O. Box 1954
> Thomasville, GA 31792
> 1-888-872-2443
> Fax: (229) 227-1752
> www.diabetestechnologies.com

Appraise A1c Diabetes Monitoring Systems. Includes postage-paid mailer. Results can be faxed, mailed, or e-mailed to patient and physician.

Matria Laboratories, Inc.
P.O. Box 2975
Shawnee Mission, KS 66201
1-888-593-2747
www.matria.com

A1c At Home. Sold by mail order and over the counter at some pharmacies. Results by fax, mail, or e-mail.

FlexSite Diagnostics, Inc.
3543 SW Corporate Pkwy
Palm City, FL 34990
1-877-212-8378
www.flexsite.com

BioSafe A1c Hemoglobin Test Kit. Kit includes postage, sold by prescription.

BioSafe Laboratories, Inc.
300 Knightsbridge
Lincolnshire, IL 60069
1-888-700-TEST
www.ebiosafe.com

A1c Now. Sold by prescription, Disposable, one-use device gives results in eight minutes.

Metrika, Inc.
510 Oakmead Parkway
Sunnyvale, CA 94085
1-877-METRIKA
www.metrika.com

Fructosamine. A lesser known glycated protein test is the fructosamine test. This test indicates average glucose over the preceding two to three weeks, so it gives a view of glucose control within a much tighter "window" than does HbA1c. Your doctor can order this test from the laboratory. A simple once-a-week home fructosamine test was briefly available on the market and may later be reintroduced by one of the large meter companies.

ONE TEST YOU CAN GIVE UP—USUALLY

We've spent most of our time here telling what you ought to do for good control. Now we'll mention something you *can* and *should* give up—urine testing. Since the diabetics we come in contact with are mostly highly motivated people who like to stay on the cutting edge of the latest diabetes therapies, we'd begun to think that nobody does urine testing anymore. But we've discovered in our reading and in conversations with diabetes educators that there are still a bunch of urine testers out there in Diabetesland.

In olden days, when the technology hadn't been developed for home blood-sugar testing, people used to test their urine in order to at least get some idea of how high their blood sugar had been because when the blood sugar is high a certain amount of sugar "spills" into the urine. This can be registered on a urine-testing tape or strip. But, as Virginia Valentine, R.N., says in *Diabetes: Type 2 and What to Do,* "Testing urine for glucose control is like driving a car using only the rear-view mirror." It doesn't show you what your blood sugar *is,* but only what it *was.* Or as Virginia puts it bluntly, "Urine testing is worthless."

When You *Should* Test Your Urine

Now, after all this haranguing about not testing your urine, there are certain times you should test it, but not to find out about your blood sugar. When you are ill or when your blood sugars are running over 250, you should test your urine for ketones. If you find you have them, it means your body is using fat for fuel, releasing fatty acids, which go into the liver, where they're converted to ketones. The presence of ketones means you're dangerously out of control and starting on the road to diabetic coma. In this case, you should contact your doctor. Usually this only applies to Type 1 diabetics.

Type 2's seldom have ketones, except when they want to and in that

FIGURE I. *How "Renal Threshold" Varies with Age**

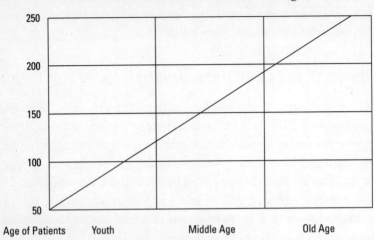

*Courtesy of Charles Weller, M.D., *Diabetes Forecast,* July/August 1978, p. 20.

case it's a happy event for them. When overweight type 2's go onto a low-carbohydrate diet (about which we'll tell you more later in the diet section), they sometimes experience what advocates of that diet call the "mild beneficial" ketosis that signals that you're losing weight. It is, they say, a normal stage of fat breakdown in a weight-loss program.

Note: Some strips are available that test for both sugar and ketones, but since you don't need the sugar test, it would be a waste of money to get that feature. The urine-testing products strictly for ketones are:

Chemstrip K
Roche Diagnostics
1-800-428-5074
www.roche.com

Ketostix Reagent Strips
Bayer Corporation, Diagnostics Division
1-800-348-8100
www.glucometer.com

➤**DiabetiLink #3** for type 1's: Improvements in Insulin and Insulin Injecting, Rationale for Multiple Shots, New Developments in Control (See p. 261)

➤**DiabetiLink #4** for type 2's: Taking Your Diabetes Seriously, Testing More than You Want to, New Developments in Control, Scared Straight (See p. 267)

THINGS TO COME

As we said previously, new equipment, products, and therapies to aid you in better diabetes control are continually appearing on the scene. It's important for you to keep up on things so that as these new products and therapies arrive, you can jump on them right away to improve your control.

You can read all about these in diabetes publications and the newspapers, but that's not where you find the *very* latest information. The really hot news is in reports you get from stockbrokers concerning new product developments in companies, developments that may cause a stock to go up (or failures, as in Imclone, that may cause it to go down). We have a few friends in stockbrokerages that keep us up to date. Thanks to their reports, we heard about the nasal spray insulin before it was common knowledge, the development of a technique for transplanting fetal islet cells, and, most recently, the encouraging research on noninvasive blood-sugar tests.

PROMISES, PROMISES

Besides the cost, a major negative of blood-sugar testing is having to stick your finger to get blood samples. This still hurts, although manufacturers of new lancing devices and testing techniques persist in promising "virtually painless testing."

This brings us to the biggest promise of them all—and the one most eagerly awaited—the noninvasive test. This means testing without sticking your finger or any other part of your anatomy to get a drop of blood. The race is on and a multitude of manufacturers are eager to be the winner, because to the winner will belong the significant spoils of selling their device along with a product that must be used with it.

GlucoWatch Biographer

One potential winner in the race may already be here: the Gluco-Watch Biographer. On March 22, 2001, the FDA announced that it was approved "for use *along with,* not as a replacement for, finger-prick blood tests to monitor glucose." (How's that for hedging their bets?) They also say that you should never used a GlucoWatch reading to change your insulin therapy—and you should always check the results against a blood sugar on a conventional meter before making insulin adjustments. (Strangely enough, the inserts in conventional meters also warn you against making insulin adjustments based on *their* readings. The legal departments are always on the job!) So far, the FDA approval of the GlucoWatch extends only to adults over eighteen years of age, and it requires a prescription.

The GlucoWatch, as you might suspect from the name, is worn on your wrist. It is not technically a blood-sugar test because what it measures is the glucose in the clear fluid underneath the surface of the skin (the interstitial fluid). It does it noninvasively using disposable sensor pads, which are snapped into the meter and attached to the skin. Each pad lasts for twelve hours. The GlucoWatch must be warmed up for three hours before you can start reading your glucose levels. You can set the GlucoWatch to sound an alarm when your blood sugars are too high or too low, and approximately every twenty minutes it automatically measures, displays, records, and stores (up to four thousand readings) your glucose levels.

One drawback of the GlucoWatch may be the cost, which hasn't yet been determined although Cygnus, the company producing the meter, estimates that it will be in the neighborhood of $350 to $450, with the sensor pads costing $4 to $5 each.

Although the GlucoWatch is still in a testing phase, reports are starting to come in on its accuracy and reliability. Michael A. Pfeifer, M.D., editor of *Diabetes Forecast,* writing in the August issue of that publication said of the GlucoWatch, "Accuracy is not quite as good as a standard meter (88 percent versus 90 percent for the standard meters) and one of every four readings may vary from actual blood glucose levels by as much as 30 percent." He also points out "one se-rious drawback," the fact that the GlucoWatch can't measure blood sugar when you're sweating. Since you could be sweating because of the heat, because you've been exercising, or *because you have low blood sugar,* Dr. Pfeifer warns, "You should always have a standard meter on hand for blood checks whenever verification is necessary."

For more information, you can call Cygnus toll free at 1-866-459-2824, or check into their website: www.glucowatch.com. You can be sure that there will eventually be information on the Web on indi-viduals' experiences with the GlucoWatch.

CGMS (Continuous Glucose Monitoring System)

Another contender (sort of) is the CGMS (continuous glucose mon-itoring system) by MiniMed. One "sort of" is that it's not really non-invasive since you have to wear an extremely fine needle (about the size of a hair) in your abdomen. Another "sort of" is that you can't read your blood sugar on it. It's designed to be read in your doctor's office. What it does is register your blood sugar every five minutes. This adds up to 288 readings a day—up to 864 readings in seventy-two hours. This can show your health-care team all the ups and downs of your blood sugar and when they occur, so they can make the appropriate adjustments in your therapy. It is as accurate as a standard meter (91 percent). Obviously this is not the noninvasive test you've been dreaming about. But stay tuned. MiniMed is plan-ning a CGMS designed for patients that is certain to be less "sort of" than the current model. Keep checking into their website, www.minimed.com/patientfam/pf_products_cgms, or call 1-800-933-3322 for further developments.

Sleep Sentry

Although the Sleep Sentry is noninvasive, it is not a meter, and you can't read your blood sugar on it. It's what you might call "a one-trick pony," but the trick is a useful one and a potential lifesaver, or at least consciousness saver and a good-night's-sleep-for-parents saver. It's a wristwatchlike device that you wear—usually at night—to signal you by beeping that you have the *symptoms* of low blood sugar: perspiration and/or a lowered skin temperature. (It can give false alarms if you're perspiring because your arm is under the covers.) The Sleep Sentry costs $349, including shipping to the United States or Canada. For more information, see the website www.sleepsentry.com, or call 1-866-270-5675.

Don't Rely on High Hopes

It's great to hear early reports of breakthroughs in diabetes, because it gives you a realistic hope that things will be better. But you shouldn't give up the available good therapies and instruments and sit around waiting for the newer and better. Most of these will take years before all the problems are worked out, they get FDA approval, and become readily available—and affordable! Some therapies and instruments, unfortunately, will never make it. So don't rush out and buy stock in every company that announces a diabetes "breakthrough." And, above all, don't do something like wait to start testing your blood sugar until you can do it without sticking your finger on one of the new machines. By the time they're actually on the market, you could have done irreparable damage from high and/or erratic blood sugars.

Don't even hold off purchasing a meter because you're waiting for the possibly better, possibly smaller, possibly cheaper one that may be just around the corner. That would be akin to never getting a car because next year's model might be improved or less expensive. No, it would be worse than that, because not having a car wouldn't be a threat to your health and well-being. It might even be healthier *not* to have a car because you'd be forced to walk more. Anyway, when it comes to meters, there are almost always advantageous trade-in possibilities for your old meter when new ones come on the scene, so you can usually be assured of being able to upgrade at very little cost.

The thing you should most especially not wait for is a cure. We all know it's coming and it may not be too far away. But don't ignore your diabetes because you figure that it will be cured before too long. A cure will do you very little good if you've neglected your diabetes therapy and developed complications. Take care of your diabetes and take care of your health so you'll be in good shape for the cure and, more important, all the while be in good shape to enjoy life!

You notice that we say, "take care of your diabetes and *take care of your health.*" They are of equal importance. Remember we're focusing here on your health as much as on your diabetes. Taking care of your health, "It's a good thing," as Martha Stewart would say. And as Mae West often attested, "Too much of a good thing can be wonderful." Climb onto the total-health bandwagon for the ride of your life, and you'll discover that they're both right.

CHAPTER 2

Stress: Public Enemy Number One

. . . .

As we mentioned previously, diabetes is becoming a nationwide epidemic with many factors contributing to it. As they say about the disease, heredity loads the gun but something else pulls the trigger. We're convinced that one of the most trigger-happy something elses in modern America is stress. There is, in fact, an increasing realization among health professionals that underlying most of our major chronic health problems, including diabetes, are the pressures and tensions and fast pace of our daily lives. We're all, as the late stressed-out singer Janis Joplin put it, "living super hyper most."

It has long been known that in those people with the genetic tendency toward the disease, diabetes can be brought on by stress—by the physical stress of pregnancy, surgery, or overweight; or by the emotional stress of something like a death in the family, a divorce, or the loss of a job. What has been ignored is the fact that stress's dirty work does not end there. Stress can also be the ruination of diabetes control on a day-to-day basis. Even worse, as Drs. David S. Schade and R. Philip Eaton reported in the November 30, 1979, issue of the *Journal of the American Medical Association,* "The most common precipitating cause of ketoacidosis [the diabetic state that can lead to coma and death] is not omission of insulin but the presence of a stress." However, no one seems to be delivering the messages clearly to diabetics or doing much of anything about giving them the tools for stress management.

The first major diabetes teaching program to give systematic instruction in stress-lowering techniques was the one at the Kansas Regional Diabetes Center in Wichita. Diana Guthrie, at that time the center's diabetes nurse specialist and the recipient of an Ames Award as the outstanding nonphysician health-care educator of the year, told us that they did a study using biofeedback to teach relaxation to diabetics with special problems like alcoholism and overweight issues. The results proved that "learning to manage stress really does cause stabilization and lowering of blood sugar." As a result, they incorporated several self-help therapies for stress reduction into their teaching program for all diabetics, and teaching programs all across the nation have followed suit.

But as so often happens in matters of diabetes care, astute diabetics have often had to figure out for themselves that control is strongly affected by stress levels. For example, we once wrote a column in *Diabetes in the News* about those aspects of diabetes that irritated June the most. We then invited readers to send us their own gripes.

One reader, Beverly Meyerheim, complained about "the continued lack of recognition . . . of the relationship of blood-sugar levels . . . to the nervous system, brain, emotions, and behavior. Stress therapy and learning new adaptive responses can be most helpful. The instruction to 'tend to your emotions' is not very explicit."

And another reader, Dale B. Pierce, after airing some of her complaints, wrote, "If I had any words for young diabetics, they would be to avoid as much stress as possible. Sometimes we try to make our bodies do as much as three or four people at once and it shows up in later life."

Some diabetics do try to do "as much as three or four people at once" just to prove that they can, just to prove they are not handicapped in any way. Even we, with our firm belief in the detrimental effects of stress, sometimes fall into this trap. We were once on a two-week book-promotion tour, appearing on radio and TV and flying to a different city each day. It was grueling and exhausting enough to kill a nondiabetic ox. June grew understandably weary and even picked up a case of food poisoning and developed a fever. It looked for a while as if she might not be able to finish the tour. "You've got to go on," Barbara kept saying as she dosed June with vitamin C. "We're always telling people that a diabetic can do *everything*. You don't want to make liars out of us!" June did go on. She never missed a show.

At the end of the tour in Boston, we called on the famous diabetologist Dr. Priscilla White, who had recently retired from Boston's Joslin Clinic. When we related this story to her with a certain amount of pride of accomplishment, Dr. White smiled wisely. "Yes, I agree," she said. "A diabetic *can* do everything. But a diabetic doesn't *have* to do everything."

A STRESS WITHIN A STRESS WITHIN A STRESS

June has always believed that diabetes itself is a tremendous stress factor. The blood-sugar swings provide the physical stress. The worry over the timing of meals, the availability of food, the fitting into your life of diabetic routines such as all the blood-sugar testing, and the awkward social problems occasioned by trying to follow your diet when dining out at a restaurant or in someone's home all contribute to emotional tensions, which, in turn, are detrimental to control.

How does stress work to undermine diabetes control? Very simply put, it's this way. Stress activates the adrenal glands to bring about the fight-or-flight response built into our systems in the days when we had to either whop a dinosaur over the head or outrun him. The adrenaline would flow, signaling an increase in blood pressure and heart rate, muscular tension, a rising of blood-cholesterol levels, and, most significant for diabetics, a release of sugar from the liver to give us the fuel for the fight or flight. After the danger was over, the adrenals would shut down, allowing our ancient ancestor to relax until the next dinosaur arrived.

Today we don't generally get into literal physical altercations, nor do we do much actual sprinting away from danger. Still, we keep triggering nature's alarm system. Because of the hectic pace of multi-tasking; tense work; a boss we're not overly fond of; problems with our spouses, children, or parents; or because of city noises hammering away in our subconscious or financial worries or a million other *ors,* we tend to live in a constant state of stress. The adrenals seldom shut down and let us relax. They continually send out the signal to the liver, and up goes the blood sugar.

Stress is hard on everyone, but at least in the case of a nondiabetic, the pancreas can jump into the fray and squirt out an extra supply of insulin. An insulin-dependent diabetic has to inject more insulin, which tends to make his or her blood sugar swing from high to low; in the case of a diet- or pill-controlled diabetic, the stress may perhaps require insulin injections.

One young-adult diabetic, who originally controlled his disease with pills, told us that when he was in college he was cramming a year of Japanese study into a six-week session and at the same time was having problems with his wife. Four weeks into this stressful period, he flunked out on the pills and had to go onto 30 units of insulin. He has been on insulin ever since.

But the most vivid personal account of how stress can put your diabetes on a roller coaster came to us from Daisy Kuhn, former professor of biology at California State University, Northridge. At the end of the college semester, when she was reading her students' masters theses under the pressure of the commencement-ceremony deadline, her insulin dosage was 38 units and she had to omit her usual bedtime snack. Still, she woke up in the morning with high blood sugar. On the other hand, as soon as the semester was over and she was home just puttering around, her insulin dosage went down to 33 units, she could have her evening snack again, and she woke up with normal or even low blood sugar.

One summer, Daisy went back to campus to help students applying for medical school. She interviewed them straight through from 1:00 P.M. to 6:00 P.M. When she got home and took her blood sugar, it was hitting the heights of 330. Later that same week she went to a conference in Asilomar, a beautiful wooded area on the Northern California coast a few miles south of Monterey. After the conference she took the weekend off just to rest and enjoy the scenery. She passed out from low blood sugar.

Daisy told us that when she puts herself under pressure by "turning on the steam," even though she's enjoying the work and feeling the exhilaration of accomplishment, she either has to forgo eating 450 calories or increase her insulin to cover that amount of calories. In other words, the blood-sugar effect of high stress in her case is almost the equivalent of eating a full meal!

Stress has other unfortunate side effects for diabetics. One diabetic told us that when she's under extreme stress, as she was recently when her husband died in an automobile accident, she just ignores her diabetes. In comparison to the problems she's trying to cope with, the diabetes doesn't seem important.

It is also true that as a result of childhood conditioning, many of us seek the comfort of food when we're nervous or upset or under pressure (a friend of ours put on fifteen pounds when she was studying for the bar exam). The increased weight causes a diabetic more physical stress—and emotional distress—creating still more diabetic problems, and so the vicious circle spins.

Now, no one living in today's world can eliminate stress entirely. You wouldn't want to even if you could, because, as stress expert Hans Selye said, "Stress is the spice of life." It is even stressful when wonderful things happen to you, which Selye calls "eustress," as opposed to *dis*tress. (The next time you win the lottery, check this out by taking your blood sugar when you get the news.)

When we went on a tour of the Hawaiian Islands with a group of diabetics, many of them reported that when they were getting ready for the trip they were so happily excited that their diabetes got out of control. Another point that Selye makes is that stress will cause a body to break down at its weakest point, just as a chain breaks at its weakest link. Your weak point obviously has to do with your body's production and/or use of insulin, so you can expect your diabetes problems to escalate in proportion to your escalating stress level.

RECOGNIZING STRESSORS

To keep your most vulnerable area from breaking down, the first step is to learn how to assess your stressors. In this section, we're going to give you some good techniques for analyzing the pressures in your life and for recognizing the body's reaction to them. Many Americans have lived with tension so long that they're totally unaware that they're tied in more knots than a macramé wall hanging. They don't even remember what it feels like to be relaxed.

Any change in your life can bring on stress, whether the change is for better or worse. A normal event that causes you to have to change or adapt to new situations—any alteration in your life that requires you to adjust—is a stressor. If too many changes are made too quickly and too frequently without enough time for recovery, you undergo a damaging stress reaction. In your case, this can mean wild blood-sugar fluctuations, and these in turn will break down your physical and psychological defenses so that you develop infections, foot and eye problems, depression, and other dismals of diabetes.

Two researchers at the University of Washington in Seattle, Thomas H. Holmes and Richard H. Rahe, devised a chart and point scale of the stressful life happenings that can bring on or exacerbate illness. To use the chart, check off events that have happened to you within the last year and then total up the score by adding up the assigned values. If your score is 150, you have a fifty-fifty chance of worsening your diabetes and/or developing some other illness. A score of over 300 indicates a 90 percent chance for illness. It's not the individual events but the cluster that causes your resistance to disease to be lowered.

You might find a direct connection between the onset of your diabetes and stress by calculating what your chances of developing an illness were according to this chart the year before you were diagnosed diabetic.

Recently, a group of psychiatrists expanded this list of life changes and classified them according to desirable and undesirable. Then they studied thirty-seven diabetics for a year or more and discovered

Social Readjustment Rating Scale

EVENT	VALUE
Death of spouse	100
Divorce	73
Marital separation	65
Jail term	63
Death of close family member	63
Personal injury or illness	53
Marriage	50
Fired from work	47
Marital reconciliation	45
Retirement	45
Change in family member's health	44
Pregnancy	40
Sexual difficulties	39
Addition to family	39
Business readjustment	39
Change in financial status	38
Death of close friend	37
Change to different line of work	36
Change in number of marital arguments	35
Mortgage or loan of more than $10,000	31
Foreclosure of mortgage or loan	30
Change in work responsibilities	29
Son or daughter leaving home	29
Trouble with in-laws	29
Outstanding personal achievement	28
Spouse begins or stops work	26
Starting or finishing school	26
Change in living conditions	25
Revision of personal habits	24
Trouble with boss	23
Change in work hours, conditions	20
Change in residence	20
Change in schools	20
Change in recreational habits	19
Change in church activities	19
Change in social activities	18
Mortgage or loan of less than $10,000	17
Change in sleeping habits	16

Social Readjustment Rating Scale (*continued*)	
EVENT	VALUE
Change in number of family gatherings	15
Change in eating habits	15
Vacation	13
Christmas season	12
Minor violation of the law	11

that there was definitely a relationship between the occurrence of life changes and adverse effects on diabetes. More significantly (and not surprisingly), they found that *undesirable* events in particular were the most detrimental for diabetics. In an article in the journal *Diabetes,* Dr. Lawrence E. Hinkle Jr. of New York Hospital pointed out that the kinds of undesirable life situations that caused the greatest adverse effect on diabetes control were either "acute conflicts with significant individuals," usually parents, husbands, wives, or children, or the threat of the loss of such a significant person.

BODY LANGUAGE

Besides monitoring your life changes for stress, you can also watch your body patterns. Our bodies give off signals when they're tense. Learn these signals and you'll know when you'd better start doing something about the tightness, tension, and anxiety you're exhibiting.

* *Breathing.* This is the best indicator of what's going on inside you, and is often the very first sign. Short and shallow breathing means tension; holding your breath means extreme tension.
* *Muscle stiffness and aching.* These reflect tightness and gripping over long periods of time. Head, neck, shoulder, and upper-back muscles are most involved. When you grip hard you often tighten your fist, hunch your shoulders, or clench your jaw.
* *Warmth.* Overworked nerves create heat; you may even perspire under too much pressure, literally breaking into a sweat.

- *Fatigue.* Anxiety and frustration cause exhaustion, even though you may be doing nothing strenuous physically. Emotion, especially bottled-up emotion, is the problem, not overwork.

BLOCK THAT STRESS

All right then, what are you to do when you find yourself assailed by too many changes and holding your breath over them? You can't become a hermit or a dropout from life. You have to and *want* to take an active part in the world, no matter how stressful that world is. Naturally, you should try to avoid any stresses that *are* avoidable. You'd no more court stress than you'd court disaster. (For a diabetic they can be the same thing.) Nor would you try to numb out the stress with drugs and alcohol. No, for all the stresses that can't be avoided (or that you don't want to avoid) what you must do is find ways—healthful ways—to diminish their adverse effects on you. After all, in most cases it is not external stress that causes your diabetic problems but your internal reaction to this stress. Incidentally, Selye says that different people can tolerate different levels of stress. Those he calls "tortoises" can comfortably handle very little stress. They need tranquillity. Those he designates "hares" thrive on stress levels that would flatten a tortoise. In fact, hares feel stressed if they don't have a certain amount of excitement—thrills and chills—in their lives. (*Note:* tortoises and hares almost invariably marry each other, thereby creating stressful stress-capacity conflicts.) But whether you're a tortoise or a hare, you have to learn how to manage stress and keep it from getting to you.

STRESS FIGHTERS

The latest analysis of the value of managing stress and the best ways of doing it appeared in an article in the January 22, 2002, *New York Times,* "Calculating the Benefits of Managing Stress" by David Tuller. This article was based on a Duke University stress management study that followed heart patients for five years. The program "emphasized the physiological effect of stress on cardiovascular disease and gave training in muscle relaxation. It also taught participants to recognize how they created stress in their lives through cognitive distortions, like mistakenly blaming themselves for bad luck."

LEARNING TO FIGHT STRESS

Cardiac patients in [this] study's stress management training were taught to identify and correct anxiety-inducing beliefs with several techniques, including:

- performing muscle relaxation and deep breathing exercises
- pausing before taking action
- writing down other possible ways to interpret events
- reviewing better ways to respond to stressful situations

Here are five examples of irrational thought patterns that produce anxiety.

STRESSOR	EXAMPLE
Catastrophizing. Exaggerating the harmful effect of something that happens to you	When your boss offers mild criticism, you're sure you'll be fired
Personalizing. Seeing yourself as the cause of a negative event	Your child fails a test, and you assume it's because you're a bad parent
All-or-nothing thinking. Reducing complex situations to absolutes	You know you're not perfect, so you must be a total loser
Overgeneralizing. Interpreting one unpleasant situation as part of an endless pattern	When you're turned down for a date, you're sure everyone will reject you
Mental filtering. Focusing on the bad while screening out the positive	You obsess about your B in history when all your other grades were As

CHAPTER 3

Diet: Theme and Variations

DIET AS HEALER, DIET AS SLAYER

Kenneth Pelletier, author of *Mind as Healer, Mind as Slayer*, considers improving the diet to be one of the basic ways of breaking a chronic stress pattern, which is detrimental to everyone's well-being. For a diabetic, diet is even more significant, because besides being a stress maker (or breaker) and a health enhancer (or detractor), diet is also an essential component of diabetes therapy. Since diet is of such primary importance for a diabetic, we'll put it in a primary position in your blueprint for building a strong body.

A THREE-LEGGED DINING TABLE

We want our diets to do three good things for us: (1) help us control our diabetes by keeping our blood sugar normal; (2) give us the proper nutrition to maintain optimum health; (3) (this is the best part) let us enjoy to the fullest the infinite and exquisite pleasures of dining. There's also one bad thing we *don't* want our diets to do—

create stress by driving us crazy as we try to figure out what diet to follow and how to do it. We'll try to help you find a diet that does the first three good things for you without a trace of the one bad one.

MY WAY

When we once went to the Hawaiian Islands on a group tour for diabetics as consultants for diabetic contingencies, a strange phenomenon occurred. Each diabetic person who had previously had intimate contact with only one diabetic—him- or herself—was thrown into a fairly close relationship with thirteen other diabetics and had an opportunity to watch carefully other diabetics' eating habits and judge them. We noticed that if a diabetic handled diet in a different way from the norm, the others on the tour would decide that the person must be goofing up or goofing off—*not doing it the right way* or "the way I do it."

Some who were diet-controlled type 2's were appalled at the way the insulin takers would sometimes be discovered lapping up a dish of macadamia-nut ice cream. When we explained that they *needed* ice cream or some other sweet to raise their blood sugar because it was too low, the diet-controlled people would look skeptical. One even suggested that these people were going out of their way to get low blood sugar just so they could eat something they weren't supposed to.

The one teenager on the trip struck terror in everyone's heart because she never seemed to sit down and eat a whole, well-balanced meal. Despite our urgings, she would pick at her plate and return most of it to the kitchen. We all eyed her nervously, wondering what was feeding her injected insulin. We kept packages of glucose tablets in our pockets, ready to pop a few into her mouth should she start turning glassy-eyed on us.

There was one woman who ate quantities of everything. She often downed sweet Hawaiian carbohydrate concoctions that would have sent the average diabetic shooting off the top of the blood-sugar scale. She wasn't overweight and appeared to be healthy. Still, we all expected to find her passed out cold in a diabetic coma with her breath giving off the fruitiness of a grape press as her bloodstream flowed with acetone, the poisonous acid price of her dietary sins.

Then it came to pass that during one of our diabetes-consultant lecture-discussions we were demonstrating how to do one's own blood-sugar testing (this was back in the bad old days before blood-sugar testing equipment and supplies were readily available). And those who seemed to be flagrant diet violators were well within the normal blood sugar range.

And the offbeat-seeming ways didn't turn out to be all that peculiar, after all. For example, we later found out that the teenager had learned from experience—several hospitalizations—that she couldn't keep in control on three normal-size meals a day. Consequently, she snacked frequently on cheese, crackers, fruit, and especially her beloved "veggies," as she called her collection of raw vegetables. She was doing what was right for her. That was how we learned that there's more than one way to feed a diabetic cat to make it sleek and glossy, with blood sugar purring along in the normal range.

MEMORIES OF THE BAD OLD DAYS—AN UNFAIR EXCHANGE

Another bad old days (pre-mid-1970s) aspect of diabetes therapy was that when you were definitely diagnosed as diabetic, the doctor—or more likely one of his office minions—pressed into your icy and trembling hand the official one-page *American Diabetes Association Exchange Lists for Meal Planning.* This divided foods into six food groups: starch/bread, meat, vegetables, fruit, milk, and fat. Based on the number of calories prescribed by your doctor, you were to select a certain number of choices of food in each group. The problem was that on this single sheet there were not many different foods to choose—only the most basic and boring ones. The gap between what June was used to eating and what was contained on the food lists was Grand Canyon–like. (In those days we were doing some writing for *Gourmet* magazine.) This can't be! And yet there it was in bold-face print: **"Eat only those foods which are on diet list."**

Only those foods? Only those prosaic staples? No more lobster? No more artichokes? No more water chestnuts? No more tortillas? No more truffles (the exotic fungus rather than the rich chocolate variety)? It must be so because not one of these had made the list.

We couldn't put up with this so we started reading and thinking and plotting to get our gastronomic lives back again. (You can read the whole pathetic adventure of June's early diabetes diet days in our book *Peripatetic Diabetic,* now out of print but available in many libraries and can be purchased used from http://www.addall.com/Rare/OOP/) or www.half.com/products/books—often for an embarrassingly low price.)

Our first hope of escape from the Valley of Dietary Despair appeared in a pamphlet published by the British Diabetic Association:

> One of the commonist misunderstandings about the diabetic diet is the mistaken impression that a diabetic can never eat certain foods. Generally speaking, there is no food a diabetic cannot include in his diet *provided that he knows and takes into account its food value.*

Aha! There's the clew—as the British would spell it. If you wander from the exchange list, you have to know *exactly* what you're eating. A home economics professor friend put us in touch with Bowes and Church's *Food Values of Portions Commonly Used.* Although this remarkable book didn't contain an analysis of truffles, it did have lobster and artichokes and water chestnuts and tortillas and, in addition, such exotics as reindeer milk and raccoon meat (both raw and cooked.) Who could ask for anything more? Well, if you insist on truffles, we think that at over $50 an ounce you could feel free to eat as many of them as anyone ever offers you. That's what June plans to do.

Our next discovery was that it's mainly carbohydrate that affects blood sugar (we checked this out with the ADA). To refresh your memory, carbohydrates are "energy foods": complex carbohydrates like bread, pasta, cereals, fruit, vegetables such as potatoes, corn, winter squash, peas, beans, etc., and those industrial strength simple sugars like sugar itself, sugarful soft drinks, candies, cakes, cookies, jam and jelly, and desserts of all kinds.

Since June had no weight problem except an inverse one, calories were of no concern to her. Proteins and fats weren't a problem either since they didn't contain enough carbohydrate to fret over and what there was fed in slowly. Therefore, all she really needed to count were the carbohydrates. Her doctor had ordered an 1,800-calorie diet composed of 180 grams of carbohydrate, 50 grams of protein, and 80 grams of fat a day Now all we had to do was figure the carbohydrate content of the various dishes she wanted to eat and keep the total under 180 grams (somewhat balanced between three meals) and she could eat virtually anything she wanted to. Life was good again. We're telling you this so you'll know that with luck and pluck and reading and thinking, you can adjust diabetes diets to you rather than you to them.

AN EXCHANGE FOR THE BETTER

Happily, those limited and inadequate Exchange Lists were revised and expanded in 1976 and again in 1986 and still again in 1995. Instead of one sheet, it grew to a thirty-two–page booklet of food choices plus information on fast foods, a list of fat-free and sugar-free or low-sugar foods, tips on label reading, and even which foods are high in sodium (marked with a red salt shaker). This booklet is available from the American Diabetes Association Publications Department (1-800-232-6733) for a mere $1.30. Of course, shipping makes it a less-than-mere $6.29, so if you can pick it up at a local ADA, office that would be a thrifty move. And the exchange list's dietary information continues to increase, finally making it as easy to follow and versatile as was purported to be back in the days when it really wasn't. Also available from the ADA is the handy, dandy sixty-four-page *Official Pocket Guide to Diabetic Exchanges.* Now virtually every diabetes cookbook and every food guide includes the exchanges for each recipe. There are also some books that are specifically aimed at expanding the exchange lists. Outstanding among these is *Exchanges for All Occasions* by Marion Franz, M.S., R.D., L.D., CDE. This covers almost every eating situation and cuisine (Jewish, Southwestern, vegetarian, etc.). It is regularly updated and available in both a standard size and pocket edition.

UP FOR THE COUNT

Much to our surprise, that carbohydrate counting method we fumbled our way into back in the early days has suddenly come into vogue. People have discovered that it's the easiest way of eating—and the most flexible—since you only have to think of one element—while, lest your dietitian have a conniption, shunning saturated fats (coconut and palm oils and other commercial shortenings, butter, and the fats found in meats, and milk). Carbohydrate counting also allows you to have much more variety in your food and thereby many more pleasurable dining experiences.

Thanks to the regulations for putting the nutritional values on food packages, it's easier than ever to know where the carbohydrates lurk and count then in your daily diet. Tip: since fiber is technically a carbohydrate, it is included in the total carbohydrate count on food labels, but you don't have to count the fiber in your daily allotment, because it is not digested. What you do is subtract the amount of fiber from the total amount of carbohydrate. That way, you'll get to squeeze in a few more carbs. Always welcome. As one T-shirt we saw put it: "I never met a carbohydrate I didn't like." For the general principles of carbohydrate counting, there is the ADA *Complete Guide to Carb Counting* by Hope Warshaw, MMSc, R.D., CDE, and Karmeen Kulkarni, M.S., R.D., CDE. Guides to the number of carbohydrates in individual foods include *Dr. Atkins' New Carbohydrate Gram Counter* by Robert C. Atkins, M.D., and *Calories and Carbohydrates* by Barbara Kraus and Marie Reilly-Pardo.

YOUR DIETARY ROAD TO SUCCESS

The most recommended and most effective way to find out which dietary road is your way is to have a consultation with a dietitian,

preferably an R.D. (registered dietitian) and a member of the AADE (American Association of Diabetes Educators). The ADA now recommends this approach, as do most doctors and dietitians specializing in diabetes. With this professional dietary guidance you can be sure you're meeting your basic nutritional needs for good health, following an eating plan that helps you keep your diabetes in control, and equally important, eating foods that you enjoy. Often a dietitian will show you how to plan your own meals with the use of the exchange lists, keeping a weather eye on the time-honored and much-revered Food Pyramid. But the basis of the Food Pyramid is starting to be nibbled away by the Healthy Eating Pyramid, developed by the Harvard School of Public Health and Harvard Medical School. (See
➤ **DiabetiLink #5:** The Healthy Eating Pyramid, p. 269)

Still at this point, the standard, government-issue Food Pyramid remains what you could call the main dietary highway, the middle-road approach. But there is a fork in the road, with the left fork leading to the HCF (high-carbohydrate and -fiber) diet and the right fork leading to the low-carbohydrate, high-protein diet. More and more people with diabetes are following the Yogi Berra admonition: "When you come to a fork in the road, take it."

HCF Diet

The high-carbohydrate, high-fiber diet (HCF) is actually an ancient diet for diabetes therapy. More than two thousand years ago, a diet rich in legumes (beans, split peas, lentils, etc.) was a common treatment regime for diabetics in India. In the 1950s, an Indian doctor, Inder Singh, put a group of his patients on a high-carbohydrate diet. He reported that the majority of them lost all symptoms of the disease and those on insulin quit taking it after three to eighteen weeks. The Japanese have used high-carbohydrate diets (white rice mainly) as standard treatment for diabetes since the early 1960s.

In this country, Dr. James Anderson of the Veterans' Administration Hospital in Lexington, Kentucky, since 1976, has published several studies showing the value of high-carbohydrate, high-fiber diets for his hospital patients. The diet he used with his hospitalized diabetic patients provided 70 percent of calories as carbohydrate, 21 percent as protein, and 9 percent as fat. On these diets, insulin doses decreased 38 percent for type 1 diabetics and 58 percent for type 2 diabetics. (He also found that these diets leveled out blood sugars of people with hypoglycemia.) Reductions in serum cholesterol values were 30 percent for type 1 and 24 percent for type 2 diabetics. Triglycerides declined 5 percent for type 1 and 4 percent for type 2.

Dr. Anderson then created a maintenance diet for use outside the hospital. This is what we now know as the HCF diet. He created his own exchanges, which are now available in his booklet *HCF Exchanges: A Sensible Plan for Healthy Eating.* His exchanges include starches (grains/vegetables like corn, peas, squash), garden vegetables, fruits, cereals, beans, milk, proteins, fats, and free vegetables. These exchanges are to be used in conjunction with his manual, *The HCF Guide Book* (Lexington, Kentucky, HCF Diabetes Foundation, 1987).

When Dr. Anderson says "carbohydrate," he means *complex* carbohydrates, or starches and very few simple sugars—only those in fruits, vegetables, and milk. And when he says fiber, he means carbohydrates packaged in their natural fibrous coating—brown rice instead of white; whole-wheat, rye, or graham flour instead of white; whole cereals like oats, bran, and cracked and shredded wheat; corn, peas, potatoes, beans, and lentils; vegetables like artichokes, bean sprouts, beets, broccoli, eggplant, kale, and squash; and fresh fruit, such as apples, bananas, melons, oranges, peaches, pears, and strawberries rather than fruit juices.

Dr. Anderson's diet gives you 30 to 60 grams of fiber a day (20 to 30 grams per 1,000 calories). Most Americans get only 12 to 20 grams a day. Both the National Academy of Sciences and the FDA now recommend that we should all eat 25 to 30 grams of fiber a day; they also believe that we should eat no more than 35 grams.

Dr. Anderson has compiled a booklet, *Plant Fiber in Foods* (Lexington, Kentucky, HCF Diabetes Foundation, 1986), which gives the fiber content in grams per serving of over 300 common foods. The analyses were made in his own laboratory.

As for protein, the diet allows only a few ounces of the leanest

Table 1: Sample Meal Plan for 1,800-Calorie Maintenance Diet

MEAL	FOOD ITEM	PORTION SIZE	WEIGHT (GRAMS)
Breakfast	Bran buds	⅔ cup	60
	Banana	½	50
	Whole-wheat toast	2 slices	46
	Skim milk	1 cup	240
	Corn-oil margarine	1 tsp	5
Morning snack	Whole-wheat muffin	1	60
Lunch	White-bean soup	1 cup	1,200
	Hash-brown potatoes	½ cup	100
	Stewed tomatoes	¾ cup	150
	Pickled beets	½ cup	100
	Fresh apple, cored	1 small	100
	Whole-wheat bread	1 slice	23
	Corn-oil margarine	2 tsp	10
Dinner	Roast beef	3 oz	90
	Baked potato	1 small	100
	Corn	½ cup	75
	Carrots	½ cup	75
	Salad: lettuce	1½ cups	100
	cucumber	1 medium	100
	Zero Dressing*	1 tbsp	15
	Peaches, water-packed	½ cup	100
	Whole-wheat muffin	1	60
	Corn-oil margarine	1 tsp	5
Evening snack	Whole-wheat muffin	1	60

*This specially prepared low-calorie dressing contains 4 calories per tablespoon.

From J. W. Anderson and Kyleen Ward, "Long-Term Effects of High-Carbohydrate, High-Fiber Diets on Glucose and Lipid Metabolism: A Preliminary Report on Patients with Diabetes," *Diabetes Care,* March/April 1978, p. 79.

meat, fish, or poultry a day. This is the hardest requirement for most people to follow. Egg yolks are taboo, as are all cheeses except the lowest in fat, like dry cottage, farmer, or hoop cheeses. Fish and poultry (skinned before cooking) are recommended. Meat choices are pretty much limited to lean beef cuts, lean pork, and well-trimmed veal and are to be used more as garnishes and flavorings for vegetables and rice dishes than as main courses.

And now we come to where the dietary belt really gets tightened: the fats. The 1,200-calorie diet has five fat exchanges and only three protein exchanges. You are getting some fat as part of your protein, though Dr. Anderson's exchanges have only 2 grams of fat, while the American Diabetes Association's (ADA) lean-meat exchanges have 3 grams. The 2,000-calorie HCF diet allows nine fat exchanges daily (and six protein exchanges). Dr. Anderson recommends cooking with Teflon pans, using Pam (a nonstick vegetable coating for pans), and eliminating oils as much as possible in baking breads and muffins. Milk exchanges are all nonfat.

This brief outline of the way the HCF diet is distinctive from the ADA diet is in no way a picture of what the day's meals are really like. In fact, the big complaint Dr. Anderson gets from his patients the first week is, "I can't eat all that food." And to help you understand why, Table 1 presents a sample day's menus for the 1,800-calorie HCF diet. Besides the foods listed, coffee, tea, and other low-calorie beverages are allowed as desired.

Eyes bulging in disbelief at the amount of carbohydrates, you are probably reacting as June first did: "This is nutritional suicide." But you're mistaken. This diet is simply a different and, for some of you, possibly a better way to handle your health and possibly your diabetes. But before you decide to "HCF it," here are some pros and cons for you to consider.

The Pros

Insulin Elimination or Reduction. We hate to even mention the idea of insulin elimination because some of you will feel that's such a pro it will outweigh any con we can come up with. But we're talking facts and here are the facts, as stated by Dr. Anderson himself:

> For lean diabetic individuals *very good* responses are likely for adults with good glycemic control using diet, oral hypoglycemic agents *or* less than 25 units of insulin daily. With HCF diets, most

of those taking oral hypoglycemic agents can discontinue them and over one-half of those taking insulin can discontinue it and maintain good glycemic control with diet and exercise. HCF diets lower serum cholesterol by 20 percent and triglycerides by 10 to 25 percent.

Good responses are likely for adults with good glycemic control using 25 to 40 units of insulin daily. Average insulin doses can be decreased about 33 percent and insulin reactions are less frequent. HCF diets lower average serum cholesterol by 20 percent and triglycerides by 10 to 25 percent.

Fair responses to HCF diets are observed for lean individuals treated with over 40 units of insulin daily, for those with a history of diabetic ketoacidoses, or for those individuals with type 1 diabetes. Reductions of insulin doses average 10 to 15 percent. Insulin reactions tend to be less frequent and glycemic control is somewhat improved. The major benefits relate to the 20 percent reduction in average serum cholesterol concentrations and the 10 to 15 percent reduction in triglycerides.

Please notice that all type 1 diabetics fall into the *Fair* responses group.

When we come to obese diabetic individuals, here is what Dr. Anderson has to say:

The major problem for the obese diabetic individual is peripheral resistance to insulin action. Giving exogenous insulin does not correct this problem. The measures that overcome peripheral resistance to insulin or increase insulin sensitivity are: weight reduction, high carbohydrate/fiber diets, exercise, and oral hypoglycemic agents (pills).

Theoretically, then, the best approach to obesity with diabetes is a high carbohydrate/fiber, weight-reducing diet combined with an exercise program. The oral hypoglycemic agents may be useful adjuncts for selected individuals.

In his clinical studies, Dr. Anderson's program resulted in 52 percent of the obese insulin-taking diabetics being taken off insulin completely.

For the most skeptical of you, we might add another comment from Dr. Anderson: "These diets have not increased insulin requirements in any patients."

We would also add that it is dangerous to change to this diet without working with your physician. Insulin dosages must be lowered cautiously and *slowly.* When starting individuals on his diet, Dr. Anderson requires that they be in control first; then he lowers the dosage by 10 percent, or 2 to 4 units.

Weight-Reduction Benefits. Most of you diabetics—some say as many as 85 percent—are the maturity-onset, noninsulin-dependent (type 2) variety and a great proportion of you can control your diabetes without using either insulin or pills. All you have to do to stay symptom-free is to lower your weight and keep it down, control your calories, and avoid concentrated sweets. If you're this kind of diabetic, the HCF diet could help you immensely, because it is an effective reducing diet.

Dr. Anderson is careful to make no wild claims for it even in this respect, however, saying conservatively, "Many of our patients are able to lose weight on these HCF diets. The secret to weight loss on these diets is to reduce total calories by cutting out sugar (sucrose) and greatly restricting the intake of all fats and oils."

You Are Never Hungry. When we talk to diabetes groups, one of the complaints we hear most frequently from type 2's who are conscientiously following a diet to lose weight is, "I'm always starved." We particularly remember a time when we were explaining the joys of the exchange lists and how you can eat almost anything if you just know what's in it and calculate your diet accordingly. One woman raised her hand and said, sadly, "I'm going to Italy and I won't be able to have pasta." "Oh, yes, indeed you can," said June with a cheerful smile. "You can have half a cup of it for your bread exchange."

"That's not enough," was the woman's terse response.

With the HCF diet, the woman could have doubled or even tripled that. Of course, she could have had only a teaspoon of oil and no cheese or cream on it . . . but that's a story for the "con" section later. In essence, though, being on the HCF diet is never having to say you're hungry, and for a diabetic with a weight problem, that's a lot not to have to say.

Lower Food Bills. The HCF diet costs about 30 percent less than the normal diet. You get a lot more vegetables, grains, and legumes for your money than you do meat, fish, and cheese. Since a great number of diabetics are in their retirement years on fixed incomes, the lower cost of food alone is a heavy plus.

A Healthier Diet. You read about it every other day. The American diet is unhealthy, primarily because it's too high in fats (particularly saturated fats) and meats and too low in complex carbohydrate and fiber. In other words, to be healthy the American diet should become the HCF diet. The low-fat–diet concept is being emphasized for all Americans and especially for diabetics, as is the low-saturated-fat idea, because fat boosts blood cholesterol and triglycerides (blood fats), both of which contribute to the cardiovascular problems to which diabetics are particularly susceptible.

But that's not the end of the fat story for diabetics. It is now thought that in overweight type 2 diabetics the problem is not lack of insulin but the inability of insulin to get into the cells, what Dr. Anderson calls "peripheral resistance to insulin." These diabetics often have abnormally *high* insulin levels in their blood. Excessive fat in the blood may well be what prevents the insulin from being used. As Dr. Anderson says, "For many diabetics, the fat in their diet is their worst enemy. Eating fat blocks the action of insulin—the body cannot burn sugar very well after a meal containing a lot of fat."

Another problem with fats is that many experts believe they make you fat. (This idea is strongly disputed by followers of the low-carbohydrate diet, as you'll see later on.) Fat is two-and-a-quarter times higher in calories than either carbohydrate or protein. Fat has 9 calories per gram while carbohydrate and protein have only 4.

What may deliver the coup de grace for fat is that all the chemical culprits of modern agriculture and pollution tend to be stored in animal fat. That makes a pretty solid case for a low-fat diet.

Moral Fiber

The high-fiber aspect of the diet is another old idea whose time has come again. Fiber was a basic component of diets of yore when refining and processing weren't in flower—or flour. Fiber is also high in the diets of primitive tribes in such places as Africa. A British physician, Dr. Denis Burkitt, helped fiber make its comeback by reporting on the low incidence among the African tribespeople of those common American problems of cardiovascular disease, cancer of the colon, diverticulosis, ulcerative colitis, varicose veins, and gallbladder disease. If fiber helps prevent all this, you can see what a total health product it is.

How about fiber and diabetes? Here's a sad tale of the South Pacific told by Dr. Denis Burkitt in a lecture reported in the June 1984 issue of *Medical Update.* On the tiny island of Nauru, everyone lived happily and healthily on a diet mainly of coconut and yams. Then they discovered that the island was covered with phosphate from the sea bird guano. It could be sold for fertilizer for so much money that the Nauruans became the second wealthiest people on earth. They immediately gave up their native diet and began importing fancy, processed low-fiber foods from Australia and New Zealand. The result is that now 30 percent of all Nauruans over the age of fifteen have diabetes.

Again we'll give Dr. Anderson the last word on the particular benefits of fiber for diabetics:

> Eating plant fibers . . . improves glucose and fat metabolism. Starches and sugars are more slowly absorbed when they are eaten as part of a high-fiber diet. Thus, the blood sugar does not go as high after a high-fiber meal as it does after low-fiber meals.
>
> Several plant fibers lower blood-cholesterol values in a dramatic fashion. Beans and oatmeal have the type of fibers that lower the

blood-cholesterol level. Our HCF diets lower the blood-cholesterol levels by an average of fifty points (50 milligrams/100 milliliters).

High-fiber diets also tend to lower blood triglycerides. Because plant fibers lower the blood fats they may be beneficial in preventing heart disease and hardening of the arteries.

More Vitamins and Minerals. The foods you eat in greatest quantity on the HCF diet are exactly the ones that are the richest in vitamins and minerals. Whole-grain bread, that great repository of B vitamins and trace elements, is another example. And, of course, the heaps of vegetables deliver even more on the vitamin and mineral line.

The Cons

Highs and Low. Now, after making it sound as if the HCF plan is possibly the Messiah of diets for all diabetics, we feel we should reveal a few flies in this all-healing ointment. In the first place, the HCF diet takes some getting used to physically. Everybody who goes on it experiences strange stomach rumblings and excessive flatulence (gas) during the adjustment period. This eventually passes—in every sense of the word—but until it does many people find it distressing.

During your adjustment period, as a diabetic you may record a few high blood sugars from the unusual amounts of carbohydrates. This is a transition stage. Later—as your insulin needs start going down—you experience frequent low blood-sugar incidents. These unpredictable highs and lows and changes are why you have to work so closely with your doctor if you embark upon the HCF diet.

Actually, the ideal way to go on the HCF diet is to spend two weeks in the hospital having your blood sugar monitored by Dr. Anderson and your body fed exactly the right meals by Beverly Sieling, his dietitian. But, since so few of us are veterans who happen to live in Lexington, Kentucky, and can be admitted to the VA hospital where both of them work, this is not a practical solution.

It's Un-American. Every diabetes book you read (including ours) and every diabetes lecture you attend make a point of insisting that you *can* live a "normal" life as a diabetic. Nevertheless, in our steak and hamburger and hot dog and pizza and ice cream culture, the HCF diet is simply not the "normal" American diet. You particularly realize this when you try to dine in restaurants or eat in fast-food chains. Meat arrives in gross hunks. When you can only eat two or three ounces of it, you wind up with more in your doggie bag than in your stomach. Fat is everywhere—sludging up the salad, drowning the vegetables, blobbed over potatoes, melting onto warm rolls, and invisibly lurking in everything. You have to ask the waiter for so many things on the side that you hardly have anything in the middle.

As for fiber, it's nonexistent. Most restaurant menus are composed of foods that have been processed to a fare-thee-well or, more accurately, fare-thee-ill. Even in health-food and vegetarian restaurants that purport to practice conscientious cookery, you can't escape the fat. It's cheese-this and nuts-that and avocado-the-other-thing.

And all diabetics already know the obstacle course of trying to keep to their diets while dining at the homes of friends. The HCF plan is possible only if you have diet-conscious friends or are most intimate with vegetarians and those in the know about nutrition.

Meat and cheese, incidentally, are what most people miss the most on the HCF diet. Meat is what too many American meals still revolve around. Cheese is many people's favorite protein, but you're restricted to the relatively fat-free varieties such as low-fat cottage cheese, ricotta, part-skim-milk mozzarella, and all the special low-fat, low-cholesterol cheeses now on the market, like *Lifetime.* Happily, many of these new low-fat cheeses are quite delicious and melt well in cooking.

Psychological Deprivation. Since the body and mind are so intimately interrelated, there can be some psychological problems associated with the HCF diet. For those who feel breakfast isn't breakfast without bacon and eggs, for example, then breakfast *isn't* breakfast and they go around feeling unsatisfied all day long. As another example, for diabetic teenagers, who have already given up so much of being dietetically one of the gang, to have to forgo the ubiquitous hamburgers, french fries, and pizza as well can become the lump of coal on top of the deprivation sundae.

No matter how healthy and slenderizing the HCF diet would be for the entire family (and it would be), it won't be easy to get them— without the goad of diabetes—to make the "sacrifices" this diet involves. And it's not easy to prepare the HCF diet for one member of the family and the "normal" diet for everyone else.

In fact, it's not easy to fix the HCF diet for anyone. It involves cooking lots of pots of beans and soups and cutting up vegetables and baking from scratch and shopping daily for fresh fruits and vegetables. Dr. Anderson himself has come to realize that, as he says, "high-fiber diets are not for everyone."

Still, it *can* be done; but if you feel your life is already unbelievably cluttered with thoughts and activities related to diabetes, then no matter how effective and revitalizing and therapeutic the HCF would be for you, it probably *isn't* for you.

If, on the other hand, you feel it *is* for you or at least *might be* for you and you want to explore its possibilities further, you can go to two websites: www.hcf-nutrition.org and www.anderson.org for more information. If you want to order some of the publications of the HCF Foundation or request a publications list, you can call the Foundation at 859-268-2020, leave a message, and they will return your call and do your bidding.

LOW-CARBOHYDRATE, HIGH-PROTEIN DIET

As the Bette Davis character in the classic movie *All About Eve* said, "Fasten your seat belts, it's going to be a bumpy night." Also a bumpy day. It will be bumpy any time the topic of the low-carb/high-protein diet for diabetics comes up. When we wrote what we thought was an even-handed consideration of the pros and cons of it in our late newsletter *The Diabetic Reader,* we were bombarded with wrath from dietitians specializing in diabetes. One dietitian cancelled her subscription, saying that her doctor had forbidden her to read it again because it raised her blood pressure too much. Another wrote, "I am a registered dietitian and diabetes educator. I find your 'publication' to be a disservice to 'people with diabetes and those who care for them' (referring to the motto of our 'publication'). The information you provide in *Diabetic Reader* is often far from accurate, and often does not reflect American Diabetes Association recommendations."

But our favorite was a phone call from a woman, undoubtedly a dietitian, who said to Barbara, "May I ask you a question?"

"Of course," Barbara cheerily replied.

"Just why are you promoting kidney failure among people with diabetes?"

What causes all this sound and fury over the low-carb diet from health-care professionals—particularly dietitians? As you can see from the illustration on page 52, for one thing, it turns the almost universally accepted Food Pyramid upside down. For another, it is, as endocrinologist Dr. Calvin Ezrin explains, because "it negates everything they have learned—and taught!—over the course of their careers. It's profoundly threatening to them."

But not all anger was directed toward us. Some of the diabetics who had failed miserably on the conventional and approved diets started experimenting with the low-carb diet. Usually they did this on their own, braving disapproval from their dietary advisers. When this diet almost immediately helped them achieve the blood-sugar control they'd been desperately seeking, sometimes for years, they were furious. "Why didn't someone tell me about this before?" They became even more furious when their dietitians continued to fight them on this "fad diet," telling them they were surely going to wreck their health if they stayed on it.

Just what is this dietary source of so much controversy and how did it erupt on the diabetes scene?

It is described in detail in *Dr. Bernstein's Diabetes Solution; A Complete Guide to Achieving Normal Blood Sugars* by Richard K. Bernstein, M.D.

Dr. Bernstein is known among his medical colleagues as the "Tartar of tight control." He is dead set against a high-carbohydrate diet because it is his belief that carbohydrates raise blood sugar as well as

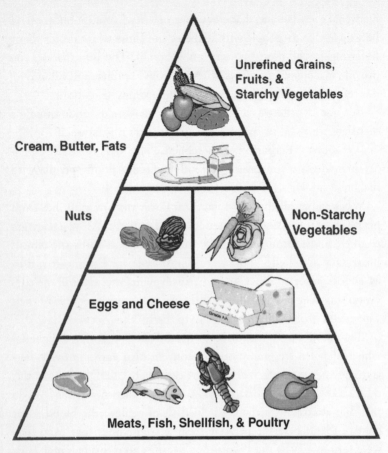

Reprinted by permission of Jeff David with special thanks to Toni-Ann Siano for the graphic representation of the pyramid.

cholesterol and triglycerides in people with diabetes. He cites studies in the late eighties that "demonstrated lower levels of blood glucose and improved blood lipids [fats] when patients were put on lower-carbohydrate, high-fat diets." His contention is that "the evidence is now overwhelming that elevated blood glucose is a major cause of high serum lipid levels and, more significantly, the major factor in high rates of various heart diseases associated with diabetes."

Dr. Bernstein has never been reluctant to go against the current. We'd even say he positively enjoys the role of iconoclast and because he does he has been responsible for several innovative breakthroughs in diabetes therapy. Diabetic himself since the age of twelve, he was always on the alert for ways to improve his therapy. In 1971 he discovered the existence of a blood-glucose monitor (Ames Eyetone). Since it was a prescription item, he had his psychiatrist wife purchase one for him and he began testing his own blood sugar on a daily basis. With the meter he devised a new self-management method that involved six blood-sugar tests a day and doses of regular (fast-acting) insulin before each meal, along with some Ultralente (long-range) insulin for long-range control instead of the conventional one shot of NPH a day.

Using his own method, he was able to keep his blood sugar within the normal range 90 percent of the time. He also discovered that protein did not raise his blood sugar after meals as fast or as much as carbohydrates, and this, too, he incorporated into his program.

Since he soon realized that in order for his discoveries to make an impact on the diabetes-therapy scene he'd have to have the right credentials, at the age of forty-five he resigned his corporate executive position and enrolled in the Albert Einstein College of Medicine, where he earned his medical degree.

We got acquainted with him back in 1976, when he was one of the 150 contributors to our *Diabetic's Sports and Exercise Book*. At that time he introduced June to blood sugar self-testing, and she gives him credit for the fact that after thirty-five years of diabetes she has no complications.

Dr. Bernstein's rationale for his diet is that carbohydrates must be kept at a minimum because they cause rapid rises in blood sugar. Protein, on the other hand, is converted much more slowly to glucose and does not cause a rapid rise. He feels that fat is safe because it has no effect on blood sugar. (For the length of time it takes different types of carbohydrates and protein to be converted to glucose during metabolism and how long it takes the glucose to disappear from the blood, see

➤**DiabetiLink #6:** Dr. Bernstein's Chart of Food Conversion to Glucose, p. 271.)

Dr. Bernstein and the patients he has trained are able to keep their blood sugars absolutely normal after eating. He does not even approve of rises of up to 150 after a meal, as many endocrinologists do. These are his guidelines for a diet that slows the rise in blood sugar after a meal:

1. Total elimination of foods that contain simple sugars.
2. Limitation of total carbohydrate intake to an amount that will not cause a postprandial (after-eating) blood-glucose rise or, in type 2's, overwork the already depleted reserve of pancreatic cells that produce insulin (beta cells).
3. Stopping eating before you feel stuffed (though there is no need to leave the table feeling hungry).

The typical carbohydrate distribution for the day's meals (examples appear in parentheses) is:

Breakfast: 6 grams of carbohydrate (¼ bagel)
Lunch: 12 grams of carbohydrate (2 cups of salad)
Dinner: 12 grams of carbohydrate (⅓ cup pasta)

Protein is whatever amount you like (for example: breakfast—2 ounces; lunch—4 ounces; dinner—6 ounces), but the amounts per meal should be consistent every day. The amount of fat can vary from meal to meal, but watch total calories if you are overweight.

As Dr. Bernstein points out, keeping track of grams of carbohydrates and ounces of protein requires far less effort than following the Exchange System. Finally, let us give you a picture of what you don't eat on Dr. Bernstein's diet—allowing, of course, for individual variations. Here is his list of foods to avoid: powdered sweeteners; most so-called diet foods and sugar-free foods (except diet sodas, sugar-free Jell-O–brand gelatin desserts, and No-Cal–brand syrups); fruits and fruit juices (including tomato and vegetable juices); desserts and pastries; milk, cream, and cottage cheese; powdered milk substitutes and coffee lighteners; snack foods (pretzels, potato chips, crackers, and so forth); candies, including sugar-free brands; cold cereals (except ½ cup puffed wheat), hot cereals; most commercially prepared soups; cooked carrots, cooked potatoes, cooked corn, beets; bread, crackers, and other flour products (some diabetics can tolerate small amounts); pancakes and waffles; cooked tomatoes, tomato paste, and tomato sauce; honey and fructose; most so-called health foods; white and brown rice; pasta and wild rice (though these may be consumed in small amounts).

So what do you eat? You eat vegetables; meat, fish, fowl, and eggs; cheeses; soy milk; nuts; zero-carbohydrate soups; yogurt; soybean flour; soybean bacon, sausages, hamburger, and steak; GG Scandinavian bran crispbread and Bran-a-crisp; coffee, tea, seltzer, mineral water, club soda, diet sodas; mustard, pepper, salt spices, herbs; table sweeteners like saccharin, aspartame, and cyclamates; zero-carbohydrate chewing gum; toasted *nori;* frozen diet-soda pops; very low-carbohydrate desserts (recipes appear in his book); alcohol in very limited amounts and of very limited kinds.

When it comes to fats, Dr. Bernstein wants his patients to minimize them, especially saturated fats. But he believes that "loading with carbohydrates will probably be more harmful in the long run than loading with fats."

As for fiber, he again goes against the mainstream. To him, fiber consumption is of no special benefit to diabetics. He claims that the haphazard use of food high in fiber can be harmful to blood-sugar control in type 1 diabetics. He acknowledges the fact that plant fiber does appear to reduce postprandial blood-sugar elevation in some diabetics who still produce part of their own insulin and in some type 2's, but that's as far as he will go in joining the high-fiber school of thought.

Dr. Bernstein is not alone in this view. Though Dr. Anderson and others have shown the many health benefits of fiber, its lowering effect on blood sugar is still debatable. Marion Franz, R.D., in "Your Fiber Guide: Understanding What Fiber Is and How It Helps," published in *Diabetes Forecast* (January 1988), wrote, "Nor is it clear . . . how reliable a tool fiber can be for helping to control blood-sugar levels in people with diabetes." Once again, the only way to see if fiber helps or hinders you is to make your own tests with high-fiber foods. For example, compare your blood sugar after a measured serving of beans with what it is after your usual carbohydrate serving at lunch and see what happens. That's the acid test.

A final consideration about the high-protein diet is its effect on the kidneys. Even high-performance athletes are being warned that increasing protein does not increase their strength or promote muscle building. Increased protein, evidence shows, has no relationship to fitness. They are also cautioned that too much protein and/or taking amino acid supplements can be harmful. It can cause long-term damage to kidneys and interfere with normal digestion of protein. This is one of the most controversial aspects of Dr. Bernstein's diet. Since diabetics are often subject to kidney problems, most dietitians cringe with horror at the high-protein level in the low-carbohydrate diet. They feel that all this protein will cause kidney problems. Dr. Bernstein disagrees. He states that the high-protein diet won't *cause* kidney problems, but if a person already has kidney trouble, then it might make the condition worse.

Physical Benefits

The obvious and greatest benefit of Dr. Bernstein's diet and method of handling diabetes is that blood sugar is normal (80 to 90 milligrams/deciliter) an overwhelming percentage of the time. This means the elimination of what he calls "the tragedy of diabetes"—such complications as blindness, kidney failure, and foot or leg amputation from gangrene. The release from fear of these so-called inevitables can't help but alleviate a formidable stress of the ongoing, unrelieved, most destructive kind for those children and adults who have tried in vain to control their blood sugars and have heretofore found no solution to their problem.

Weight Loss

Since people with type 2 diabetes often need to lose weight for diabetes control and general health, that's another area where a low-carb diet can help. Despite all of the "fat makes you fat" information you've been bombarded with over the years, the low-carb proponents insist that it ain't so. They maintain it's the carbohydrates that do the deed because they cause the pancreas to release more insulin and insulin is a powerful fat-building hormone.

Off to a Fast Start on Blood-Sugar Control

In *Diabetes Type 2 and What to Do,* Virginia Valentine, R.N., describes the "Fast Fast" that she uses to help her type 2 patients get their blood sugars under control quickly or to get them off medications. She explains that it's not a total fast, merely a fast from carbohydrates. After the situation is under control, she has them gradually start adding one carbohydrate at a time to see the effect increasing carbohydrate has on their blood sugars.

An Imprudent Diet

For born-again diet freaks as we admit to having been from time to time in our careers, this diet, with its high protein and fat and low carbohydrate and fiber, seems downright unhealthy. Indeed, in most respects it's the direct opposite of the recommendations of the American Diabetes Association, the American Heart Association, the American Cancer Association, and the National Research Council.

As we previously mentioned, the high-protein diet is particularly inadvisable for those who already have kidney damage. Cookbooks for diabetics on dialysis all feature low-protein diets (below 50 grams a day) because protein makes the kidneys work harder. Kidney function also declines with age, and this means that older people should, if anything, lower the amount of protein they eat.

And one more caveat: excess protein can cause you to lose calcium and therefore promote bone loss. This is particularly inadvisable for post-menopausal women who are already at risk for osteoporosis. In that case, calcium supplements are recommended.

Nemesis of All Vegetarians

If a vegetarian gets it into his/her head to follow the low-carb diet, even the most enthusiastic low-carb supporters admit that it can't be done. And it's as we once read on a sign in a Dublin watchmaker's shop: "If it can't be done it won't be done." If, however, you cleverly figure out a way to do it, please let us know and we'll spread the word.

Dr. Bernstein Alone No More

Gradually, other diabetes health-care professionals and bariatricians (physicians specializing in weight loss) began pitching their tents on Dr. Bernstein's low-carb campground. Some books they have written on the benefits of the low-carb diet include:

> *Protein Power* by Michael Eades, M.D., and Mary Dan Eades, M.D., emphasizes weight reduction.
> *The Type II Diabetes Diet Book* by Calvin Ezrin, M.D., and Robert E. Kowalski is directed to diabetics who are at least 20 percent overweight. Unlike some of the other low-carb manuals, he restricts fat.
> *The Schwarzbein Principle: The Truth About Weight Loss, Health, and Aging* by Diana Schwarzbein, M.D., is based on her work with insulin-resistant type 2's when she discovered that conventional diets made their condition worse. This caused her to experiment with and ultimately embrace low-carb, higher-fat diets with great success.

And of course there are all the much-maligned (by health-care professionals) books by the late Robert Atkins, M.D., which you will find on virtually every best-seller list. (His books deal with weight loss and the principles of the diet. Not particularly aimed at diabetics.)

In our *Diabetic's Book: All Your Questions Answered,* we have included a supplement on the low-carb diet ("The Dietary Court of Last Resort"). In this we tell our adventures thereon, give tips on how to do it, and present success stories of happy low-carbers.

Check into Dean Esmay on the Web and read his dietary odyssey from high-carbohydrate, low-fat to low-carbohydrate diet. Follow his link to "The World's Biggest Fad Diet" (surprise, the fad is not the low-carb diet but the high-carb, low-fat one).

The most unexpected new supporter (with qualifications) of the low-carb diet is Dr. Julian Whitaker, author of the high-carbohydrate/

low-fat diet advocating book *Reversing Diabetes.* In the January 1998 issue of his *Health and Healing* newsletter, he forthrightly states:

> When with good reason, it becomes necessary for one to separate from a dogma that one has long supported, it is best to go ahead, do it, and get it over with. For years I have advocated a diet very high in complex carbohydrates. While I maintain my stance on the deleterious effects of excessive fats, new research has convinced me that excessive carbohydrates pose similar risks.

How's that for candor, character, and courage!

Joy to the World of the Low-Carb Diet

At the annual meeting of the American Association of Diabetes Educators in Orlando, Florida, in August 1999, we were privileged to attend a presentation with the title *Lower Carbohydrate Diets in Diabetes Management: Help or Hype?* by Joy Pape, R.N., BSN, CDE, CETN. And we do mean privileged, because there was a huge line of people clamoring to get in—a bigger crowd than any we'd seen at the conference. Luckily we made it inside and even got seats. Others had to lean against the wall.

This gives an indication of the interest among health-care professionals in this diet. Probably most of those in attendance thought as we did. "Ho-hum here comes another health professional shooting down the low-carb diet as unsound, unhealthy, and unacceptable, and espousing the tried-and-true low-fat, high-complex carbohydrate one. Been there, heard that."

Boy, were we wrong! What we heard was a thoroughly professional, well-researched, completely balanced presentation of the current low-carb diet plans: Dr. Atkins's *New Diet Revolution;* Dr. Bernstein's *Diabetes Solution;* Drs. Michael and Mary Eades's *Protein Power;* Dr. Diana Schwarzbein's *The Schwarzbein Principle;* Leighton and colleagues' *Sugarbusters!;* and Dr. Barry Sears's *The Zone.*

To show Pape's dedication to discovering how effective these diets were in diabetes therapy, she visited—at her own expense—the offices of the doctors espousing these diets. This wasn't just a casual or social visit. She questioned the doctors, interviewed their patients, and even examined the patients' charts. The results of her research are clearly not the much-maligned "anecdotal evidence" that people accuse all the reports of success on the low-carb diet of being.

While Pape certainly doesn't imply that the low-carb diet is right for everyone, her conclusion is that you can't ignore the fact that there are patients who are doing better on this diet than they were doing before. Her reasonable suggestion to the AADE members was that they should learn more about the diet and give their patients a choice. (And, we might add, if they don't give patients a choice, increasingly empowered as they are becoming, they're very likely to make that choice on their own.)

After the talk, Pape was surrounded by people congratulating her, asking questions, and giving, in a nonhostile way, their reasons for fearing the diet. (Overheard from one of the dietitians in the group talking to her: "If it turns out you're right and we're wrong we're sure going to be embarrassed.")

There's an axiom told to medical students: "Never be the first nor the last to accept a new therapy." It's too late for diabetes health-care professionals to be the first to accept the low-carb diet, so they're safe there, but it might be wise for them to become at least somewhat more knowledgeable and accepting of the lower-carb diet, lest they be the last.

If you want to hear everything Joy Pape said in her memorable conference session, you can order a complete audiotape of it from:

CONVENTION CASSETTES
  1-800-776-5454
  74923 Hovley Lane East
  Suite 250
  Palm Desert, CA 92260
  Ask for tape: T13.
  Cost $11.00 + $3.50 shipping

Times They Are A-Changing

Another nail in the low-fat, high-carbohydrate dietary coffin was hammered down in the July 7, 2002, issue of the *New York Times Magazine:* "What If It's All Been a Big Fat Lie?" by Gary Taubes, who summed it up with, "At the very moment that the government started telling Americans to eat less fat, we got fatter. The truths about why we gain weight and why it is so hard to lose it just might might turn out to be much different from what we have been led to think."

THE G. I. (GLYCEMIC INDEX) JIVE—FINE-TUNING YOUR DIET

There is a story—possibly apocryphal—about how orange juice came to be the classic treatment for insulin reactions. In Canada, back when Banting and Best were conducting their initial experiments with insulin, their first patient was walking home after having had his insulin shot. He started to feel Really Strange and staggered to the door of the nearest house.

The woman answering the door said, "My goodness, young man, you look terrible! Come in and sit down. I'll give you a glass of orange juice." He soon felt better. Thus was the tradition born.

The Carbohydrate Glycemic Index based on 1981 research by Dr. David Jenkins of the University of Toronto is a gauge of how high and how fast individual carbohydrate foods raise the blood sugar. It does this by comparing the way carbohydrate foods raise blood sugar with the way straight glucose raises it. Glucose, the form of sugar in the blood, is assigned an index number of 100.

Generally speaking, for a diabetic a low (slow-releasing) Glycemic Index food is preferred to a high (fast-releasing) Glycemic Index food. The following chart shows the Glycemic Index of some foods that have been tested. Looking at this, you can see that orange juice isn't by any means the fastest food treatment for low blood sugar. Instant potatoes would be faster; so would corn flakes and parsnips and carrots. Since all of these are a little hard to carry around, it's best to stick to glucose tablets.

Glycemic Index

SIMPLE SUGARS

Fructose—20	Honey—87
Sucrose—59	Glucose—100

FRUITS

Apples—39	Bananas—62
Oranges—40	Raisins—64
Orange juice—48	

STARCHY VEGETABLES

Sweet potatoes—48	Instant potatoes—80
Yams—51	Carrots—92
Beets—64	Parsnips—97
White potatoes—70	

DAIRY PRODUCTS

Skim milk—32	Ice cream—36
Whole milk—34	Yogurt—36

LEGUMES

Soybeans—15	Garbanzos—36
Lentils—29	Lima beans—40
Kidney beans—29	Baked beans—40
Black-eyed peas—33	Frozen peas—51

PASTA, CORN, RICE, BREAD

Whole-wheat pasta—42	White bread—69
White pasta—50	Whole-wheat bread—72
Sweet corn—59	White rice—72
Brown rice—66	

BREAKFAST CEREALS

Oatmeal—49	Shredded wheat—67
All-Bran—5	Cornflakes—80
Swiss Muesli—66	

MISCELLANEOUS

Peanuts—13	Sponge cake—46
Sausages—28	Potato chips—51
Fish sticks—38	Mars bars—68
Tomato soup—38	

The Glycemic Index isn't a whole way of diabetes eating but it is an excellent way of deciding which foods to select when you don't want to run up your blood sugar, or when you *do*.

The drawback of the G.I. has always been that so few foods were analyzed—only forty-seven in the original list. Everyone kept wishing for more research on more foods. Now those wishes have come true with three books and one website:

Note: Most glycemic index numbers use glucose as a standard (100), although some use white bread. Rick Mendosa, who always leaves no diabetes stone unturned in his research and reportage, gives you both on his website. M. Montignac, maverick Frenchman that he is, uses maltose (which is actually even sweeter than glucose) as his standard.

A good book is *The Glucose Revolution; The Authoritative Guide to the Glycemic Index,* by a group of Australian and Canadian nutrition experts (including two M.D.s and a Ph.D.) These authors' thesis is that watching carbohydrate consumption is the key to good health and they show you via an expanded G.I. list of 430 foods which carbohydrates to choose. There are fifty recipes with their nutritional counts as well as their G.I. rating.

Sugar Busters; Cut Sugar to Trim Fat by H. Leighton Steward, Sam S. Andrews, M.D., Morrison C. Bethea, M.D., and Luis A. Balart, M.D., is designed as a weight-reduction plan. This way of eating is summarized in the introduction as "lean meats, chicken and fish, fresh vegetables, fresh fruit, the right low-insulin–producing carbohydrates (those low on the G.I.), and even red wine. This book expands the G.I. list to one hundred items.

Dine Out and Lose Weight is written by Frenchman M. Montignac and translated into English. It has the same principle as American low-carb diet books: "It's not the fat you eat that runs up your weight, it's the carbohydrates." Although the book is serious and can help you lose weight and lower blood sugars, it is also fun to read and easy to follow. You only eat from his list of "good" carbohydrates (those low on the Glycemic Index) and abstain from his list of "bad" carbohydrates (those high on the list.) Montignac's G.I. list is different from the American one and so provides a useful expansion to higher realms of gastronomy. As you would expect from a Frenchman, Montignac is very big on the benefits of drinking wine, citing his mother from Bordeaux, who lived until the age of 102: "She hated water and only drank red wine." This prescription was also followed by Antonio Todde, an Italian shepherd who held the Guinness record for longevity when he died just shy of his 113th birthday. He advised, "Just love your brother and drink a good glass of red wine every day."

Rick Mendosa's Glycemic Index websites (www.mendosa.com/gi.htm and www.mendosa.com/gilists.htm) are expanded lists containing a hefty three hundred items. Warning: once you discover these and Rick's other many and varied websites and links, you may never be able to tear yourself away. They are treasure troves of reliable diabetes information.

IF THE SHOE DOESN'T FIT, DON'T WEAR IT.

Once, after we had given a diabetes talk, a woman approached Barbara and asked, "How many pieces of chicken can my husband eat?" Barbara launched into a mini-lecture on how that was dependent on his weight, his daily caloric allotment, his activity level, his medication, etc., etc. The woman looked at Barbara suspiciously as if she thought she was deliberately holding back important information. Not giving up she gestured toward June and demanded, "How many pieces of chicken can *she* eat?"

We're all different and just as you can't try to fit your feet into someone else's shoes, so you can't go whole hog onto someone else's diet. If it's right for them, it's probably not going to be exactly right for you. That being said, just so you'll know we're not holding out on you, basically this is what June does:

- She counts her carbohydrates and generally follows a low-carb diet.
- She eats more fruit than is recommended on most low-carb diets.

- She leans toward fruit and vegetables that have the most fiber (raspberries, pears, strawberries, peas, corn, broccoli, Brussels sprouts, raw carrots), the better to avoid the constipation that can go with a low-carb diet.
- She keeps the Glycemic Index in the back of her mind and selects the foods that will either raise her blood sugar faster or slower, depending on her blood sugar at the time.
- She selects monounsaturated fats (olive oil, avocado oil, macadamia-nut oil, peanut oil, etc.) over polyunsaturated ones and avoids hydrogenated fats and tropical oils (coconut, palm kernel, and palm) as best she can. True confession: she eats butter, but in moderation.
- Although she does eat meat, she prefers fish, chicken, and tofu.
- She eats eggs and they have not done bad things to her cholesterol, which is always well within the normal range.

But the most important thing she does is that she's always on the lookout for dietary changes that might be beneficial. Over the years she's tried the HCF diet with some success and the mainstream diet as well. One interesting thing we've noticed is that almost any diet works well at first, when you're most meticulous and most enthusiastic about it, then as time goes by and you let down and possibly become bored by it, the effectiveness diminishes.

As June did, you have to find the diet that works for you for the long haul, and, after you've found it, keep looking for something even better down the line. Just like life, a diet is not a destination, but a journey.

CHAPTER 4

Diet: Cautionary Notes and Encouraging Words

No matter which diet plan or combination of plans you elect to follow, there are certain basic principles of dietary health that apply to all diabetics. In fact, most of these apply in large measure to all non-diabetics as well. Therefore, if you can convince your family members and friends to join you in your general dietary-improvement plan, you'll be giving them a tremendous gift of well-being. You'll also be helping yourself because it's a lot less difficult to make changes for the better in your diet if those around you aren't chomping on those health underminers we all know and love.

But just what *are* the principles of dietary health? You constantly read about them in newspapers, magazines, and books and hear about them on the radio and see and hear about them on TV. Your friends are also generous in passing along nutritional advice. But the problem is that half of the information that comes your way turns out to be misinformation the following week. In *The Diabetic Reader* we had a column called "The Fickle Finger of Food Facts; In What Strange New Direction Is It Pointing Now?" This duplicitous digit kept constantly changing, pointing you away from this food toward that food, and the next month sending you in the dead opposite direction. As Frank Sponitz, writer for the *X-Files* said:

> I'll tell you what I think has done the greatest damage to science: these studies on things like coffee. Or red meat. Back and forth and back and forth every couple of weeks it's in the newspaper. And people finally just say forget it.

But the trouble is we can't forget it. We have to pay attention to what has been called "the most intimate consumer product"—the food and drink we consume. These actually become parts of our bodies, for better or for worse. So to try to help you make it for better, we'll do our best to fairly present the current dogma of nutritional "experts" along with the conflicting fickle-finger beliefs of other "experts."

THREE FOR THE ROAD TO OBLIVION

In Western movies you can always tell the good guys because they wear the white hats. In your diet, it doesn't work that way. Three of the worst culprits who are out to gun down your health are white as the driven snow—sugar, salt, and white flour.

Bitter Sweets

It should give you some measure of comfort to know that even if you weren't a diabetic you should shun sugar as much as you have to because you are. In fact, sugar is so bad for everyone that we've heard it said if sugar were just discovered today the FDA would have to ban it because of its many detrimental effects on health.

If you want to turn yourself off sugar so completely that you shriek in terror when you pass a sugar display in the supermarket and recoil from a candy bar as if from a viper, read *Sugar Blues* by William Dufty. He blames $C_{12}H_{22}O_{11}$—the simple sugar called sucrose—for every woe and evil of humankind, including acne, menstrual cramps, cancer, depression, alcoholism, ulcers, schizophrenia, and the decline and fall of all the major civilizations in the history of the world.

Dufty, of course, is a fanatic, but even nonfanatics agree that sugar makes you fat, sugar gives you cavities, sugar raises your blood pressure, sugar increases your chances of blood-clotting problems in the veins, sugar depletes your B vitamins, and sugar ups your triglycerides. On top of all that, sugar is addictive (worse than opium and its derivatives, opines Dufty). It has been called by some the "alcoholism of children."

One secret of business success is to "find something you can make for a nickel, sell for a dollar, and is habit-forming." A lot of manufacturers of sweet products have discovered this secret. They are flailing us with advertising about their sugar-shot merchandise, and they're putting sugar in almost everything these days. That's why it's so tough to avoid sugar in our society. Sugar is such an accepted, even approved, additive in foods that it's actually illegal to label a product ketchup if it doesn't contain sugar. (The Trader Joe's chain markets its own brand of "ketchup," which is sugar-free. They have to call it "Ketchy" to get around the law.) Apparently, the ketchup producers aren't required to call sugar by name, however. On one label we saw it euphemized to "natural sweetener."

As a diabetic, you have the advantage of not being able to consume the quantities of sugar that most people thoughtlessly load up on. These quantities average out to 500 calories of sugar per person *every day.* Teenagers top even that. They consume almost 10,500 calories (close to three pounds!) of sugar a week. For diabetics, the American Diabetes Association now approves of up to one teaspoon of sugar per reasonable serving of food. The maximum number of teaspoons per day depends on personal calorie allotment. This sugar is allowable only combined with food, and only if your blood sugar is in control.

Nutritive Sweeteners

The term nutritive sweeteners is an oxymoron because they are far from nutritious. They are called that because they contain calories and carbohydrates and, as such, must be counted in your diet because they will raise your blood sugar. Huddled in the nutritive-sweetener tent along with the most common sucrose are fructose, glucose (aka dextrose), sorbitol, and mannitol.

The Sweet Alternatives

Many diabetics turn their lives into an unending quest for sweets that don't count—sweets that don't cause damage either diabetically or otherwise. As a homely philosopher has said, "There's no such thing as a free lunch"—and there's no such thing as a free sweetener. Although the so-called "nonnutritive" sweeteners are free in that they don't have calories, they do have other problems, especially if you're an overindulging mouse or rat.

Cyclamates

These came on the scene in the 1950s and remained a popular favorite until they were fickle-fingered and placed on the forbidden list in 1969. The reason was that when huge quantities (500 times the recommended maximum amount approved for human consumption) of it were fed to laboratory rats, it sometimes—very occasionally—caused bladder cancer. We're not going to debate here whether cyclamates will or will not cause cancer in humans just because those occasional rats developed it. But no matter whether cyclamates deserve their ban, they're gone until the manufacturer gets the re-approval, which it is seeking. They are still readily available in many countries including Canada, where Americans have been known to border-hop to purchase their sugar substitute of choice.

Saccharin (Brand Names: Sugar Twin, Sweet 'n Low, Sucaryl)

Some experts as well as nonexpert consumers believe that saccharin, rather than cyclamates, should have been the one banned. After all it, too, was known to cause bladder cancer in laboratory rats and mice when they were fed the human equivalent of 800 saccharin-sweetened soft drinks. Plus it is banned in more countries than cyclamates. On top of that, cyclamates just taste better (some feel saccharin has a metallic taste), if that counts for anything. Even so, it has been under the gun since 1977, but Congress keeps delaying its ban and saccharin keeps on keeping on as it has been doing since its introduction back in 1879. For a while it was required to carry a warning label, but that requirement was lifted in 2000, so it appears to be home free. It doesn't break down with heat and can be used in baking and cooking.

Aspartame *(NutraSweet)*

Aspartame is now used in an almost endless array of commercial products, from cereals to soft drinks, and the list keeps expanding. Its drawback is that it can't be used in cooking, as it loses its sweetness when heated. It can be added only after cooking. Another problem is that there have been rumblings about its safety. People with PKU (phenylketonuria)—a rare inherited metabolic disease in which you have to restrict intake of phenylalanine—have to avoid aspartame since it contains phenylalanine. The FDA has ruled that all products containing aspartame must carry a warning. The *FDA Consumer* of May 1994 also said that those with advanced liver disease and pregnant women with high levels of phenylalanine in their blood should avoid aspartame products. (Note: If you surf the Internet under the heading "Aspartame," you'll find a list of all the things that aspartame is supposed to cause that is even more wild and wooly than Dufty's inveighings against sugar.)

Acesulfame-K—*also called* Ace-K *(Sunette, Sweet One)*

Ace-K's advantage is that you can cook with it, although it does not have the volume or texture of sugar (important in baking). So far there have been no reports of rodent bladder cancer or other life-threatening conditions caused by this product.

Sucralose *(Splenda)*

The newest kid on the sugar substitute block, but you'll be hearing a lot about it since it has the marketing muscle of Johnson and Johnson behind it. It can be used in cooking and many think that—hot or cold—it has a more sugarlike taste than the others.

Isomalt-Acesulfame-K-Aspertame *(DiabetiSweet)*

This three-way product takes pride in what it *doesn't* have: sucrose, fructose, dextrose, maltodextrin, sodium, saccharin, or bitter aftertaste. It *does* have a granulated texture similar to sugar and it can be used for baking since it's stable in heat. Since this is less well-known than the other sweeteners, for more information on it you can call 1-800-899-3116 or visit their website, www.diabeticproducts.com.

Nutritive But Nice

Four substances sometimes touted as ideal sweeteners for diabetics are the nutritive sugar substances fructose, HSH, and the sugar alcohols sorbitol and mannitol. HSH (hydrogenated starch hydrolysate) is chemically the same as sorbitol. Their advantage over cyclamates, saccharin, and aspartame is that they have not been found to cause cancer in mouse bladders or seizures in people. These sweeteners also have the advantage of acting more like table sugar (sucrose) in cooking and baking. And they don't have a bitter aftertaste.

Another advantage of these for diabetics is that they are absorbed more slowly, and in the first stages of metabolization they do not require insulin. Because of this, they don't cause blood sugar to rise as rapidly after eating. (Caution: fructose will raise your blood sugar exactly as sugar does, if your blood sugar is already high!) They also seem to be less inclined to raise cholesterol and triglyceride levels than table sugar.

A disadvantage of the sugar alcohols is that in anything other than very small amounts they can cause diarrhea—not a happy event for anyone, but especially hazardous for a diabetic. According to the manufacturers of products containing HSH, it does not have as pronounced a laxative effect.

One that you might consider incorporating in your diet is fructose. Because it's one and a half times sweeter than sugar and three times sweeter than sorbitol you can use less of it for the same sweetness. Also, it *is* a natural product. In England it's called "fruit sugar" and the British Diabetic Association recommends it as the ideal cooking sweetener for diabetics. In fact, in England and the rest of Europe, it really is made from fruit, while in the United States it is made from corn. Although chemically fructose is the same in both varieties, some people claim there is a taste difference. You can purchase fructose in liquid or granular form. It has virtually the same calorie count as sugar, about 110 calories an ounce.

Not to overdo the virtues of fructose, let us point out that it has been accused of raising triglycerides and, although it is considered a fruit exchange, it is nevertheless one without the fiber and nutritive advantages of fruit. A tablespoon of fructose does not seem like a good trade for a fresh, juicy peach or ten large, sweet cherries or a small, crunchy apple. Fructose, in short, is not the free lunch you've been looking for.

What is a diabetic to do, then, to satisfy the sweet tooth that some diabetics seem to have? Rather than trying to satisfy it, we think you should just yank the rotten rascal out by the roots. Get yourself to the point where you no longer like excessively sweet things. Change your taste.

It can be done. In her pre-diabetic days, June was as hooked on her midmorning sweet roll, her Sunday pancakes and syrup as anybody. But gradually over the years her taste for sweet things, except for the natural sweetness of fruit, has left her. It took no tremendous strength of character on her part. It just happened. Now she has about one artificially sweetened soda every six months, if that. She puts fresh fruit and/or cinnamon on cereal, never sugar or artificial sweeteners. When she occasionally wants a little jam for her home-baked oat bran muffins, she uses one of the preserves or jellies that are "low sugar" or made totally of fruit. (Check the label and get the one with the lowest carbohydrate.)

If you can keep yourself from being obsessed by your "great loss" of sweets, from constantly regretting the long-gone pie à la mode, you'll probably find it wasn't such a great loss after all. You'll actually begin to discover subtle nuances of flavors that were previously buried by overloads of sugar or artificial sweeteners.

Sweet 'n Low Blow and Equal

Those little pink and blue packets you find on restaurant tables with the sugar are not as innocent as they look. The redoubtable Dr. Richard K. Bernstein has pointed out that if you take a magnifying glass and read the list of ingredients in either Sweet 'n Low or Equal, you'll find that dextrose (glucose) is the leading ingredient. Does this mean you should avoid them, even though they're supposedly for dieters and diabetics? Diabetic diabetes dietitian Meg Gaekle says one or two won't hurt you. The dextrose is there only to provide bulk and there is too little of it to be concerned if you limit yourself to a small amount in your coffee or tea. This does make a question pop into mind: How then can these be called sugar substitutes, considering what they contain?

This product and others can be designated as sugar-free or sugar substitutes because in the United States the food-labeling laws identify sugar as sucrose. Glucose, fructose, maltose, ribose, mannose, etc., are not legally sugar.

You can see from this how many "sugar-free" products are loaded with things that are sugar for all intents and purposes, except legal ones. You have to be very astute in your label reading: keep an eye out for names like xylose, mannose, dextrose, glucose, sucrose, fructose, sorbitol, mannitol, xylitol, etc. And while you're at it, keep an eye out for honey. It's as diabetically detrimental as any of the others no matter how the health-food addicts strum its praises on their guitars.

Dietetic Foods

Just as many diabetics erroneously believe sweeteners like fructose and sorbitol need not be counted on their diet, they also have the notion that special dietetic foods can be ingested as freely as water and air. Not so! "Dietetic," when used on food labels, has a very precise, ADA-defined meaning. To quote the ADA Exchange Lists, "It means that something has been changed or replaced. It may have less salt, less fat, or less sugar. It does not mean that the food is sugar-free or calorie-free."

Monetarily they are a long way from free. In fact, they sometimes cost twice what their regular nondietetic counterparts cost. And what do you get for these megaprices? A study by Irene M. Wunschel and Bagher M. Sheikholislam of the University of California at Davis revealed that while the amount of carbohydrates in dietetic candy and cookies was less than in regular candy and cookies, the calories and fat were greater. Preserves, syrups, puddings, gelatin, and ice cream rated better in terms of reducing the things a diabetic needs reduced (calories, carbohydrates, fats), but the price differential was significantly greater. Their conclusion was, "In most instances, the consumer receives little or no nutritional benefit from the higher cost of the dietetic product. Indeed, the use of dietetic products may replace foods with important nutrient content. . . . The most beneficial intake is one derived from a wide variety of ordinary foods."

The ADA considers only some dietetic foods useful for diabetics: "Those that contain 20 calories or less per serving may be eaten up to three times a day as free food."

Shaking Salt

Dr. Andrew Lewin, deputy director of the Hypertension Detection Program at Cedars-Sinai Medical Center in Los Angeles and director of Pressure Partners, a medical program to help patients lower their blood pressure, believes that most Americans are salt addicts, consuming 10 to 20 grams of sodium per day. Though health professionals can't agree on the exact amount, the maximum safe level is more like 2 or 3 grams a day. (A level teaspoon of salt contains 2.3 grams of sodium; a four-ounce bag of potato chips has about 1 gram.)

So what if we use too much salt? So a lot. It contributes to high blood pressure, or hypertension, as it's medically called. Studies have revealed that cultures in which the most salt is consumed have the highest rate of hypertension, which is a result of increased water retention in the body. Too much salt also causes swelling of the tissues (edema), which decreases the amount of oxygen they receive, and this in turn can bring a variety of problems associated with circulation.

The "so what" of all this for diabetics is pretty obvious. The problems salt aggravates are many of the same problems diabetes aggravates. Nobody needs double aggravation.

Type 2 diabetics who are moving toward (or already into) the high-incidence-of-hypertension years have a particular need to cut back on their salt. But it's a good idea for young diabetics to begin with the basic good-health habit of salt reduction at an early age on the ounce-of-prevention theory. Dr. Lewin believes reducing salt intake will possibly prevent high blood pressure in susceptible persons.

Since everyone under stress is advised to reduce salt in order to avoid the physical stress of water retention, it is only logical that every diabetic who carries around the built-in stresses of this disease wouldn't want to add to them with a salt load. If you want to reduce the salt in your diet, here are some tips from Pressure Partners.

1. Learn to distinguish those foods that are high or low in sodium.
2. Read labels carefully to determine the sodium content of processed foods.
3. Avoid processed foods, since they generally contain relatively higher amounts of sodium than their natural or *frozen* counterparts.
4. Avoid snack foods and restaurant fast foods, which are high in sodium, particularly if you know you have high blood pressure.
5. Find a market that stocks low-sodium products if you have been placed on a sodium-restricted diet.
6. Bring out the natural flavor of foods without using table salt by adding lemon juice, curry powder, herbs, spices, wines, and fruit juices.
7. Use onion and garlic to perk up flavors naturally.
8. Develop your own spice shaker to use at the table in lieu of salt. The shaker may contain onion powder, garlic powder, pa-

prika, pepper, and mixed Italian herbs, or you can create your own blend.

Cutting back on salt is one of the easier cutbacks. We discovered this from talking to a dietitian. She said that in her work she was always telling people to take things they enjoyed out of their diets and telling them there was nothing to it, so she decided to try a little self-restricting herself. Since she knew that no one needs additional salt (you get more than you need on a normal diet), she put away her salt shaker and salted nothing at the table. In a few weeks she didn't miss the additional salt at all.

Speaking of not salting at the table, that's particularly important when dining out. In the better restaurants, the chef is mortally wounded when people pour salt over their dishes, which he considers already perfectly seasoned. Some don't even put salt on the table. Here's another tip. If you're in the running for an important job and the powers that hire take you out to lunch or dinner, according to an article about job interviews, one thing they watch out for is if you salt before tasting the food. That indicates a person who doesn't evaluate situations before taking action—just the kind of person they don't want. (It also indicates you're not a person with a sophisticated palate and would be unable to impress prospective clients you entertain.)

Actually, by giving up salt at the table you may make it unnecessary to have to give it up completely in later years, adding the restriction of a totally sodium-free diet to your already restricted diabetic diet. It's a matter of practicing moderation in order to keep from having to practice abstention.

There have been some recent reports suggesting that sodium may not directly contribute to high blood pressure. Nevertheless, most experts still agree that the 60 million Americans who have high blood pressure should cut back on sodium. Consequently, until evidence to the contrary is clearer, we'll personally continue to consider sodium a dietary criminal; at least it commits a misdemeanor if not a felony.

But Richard K. Bernstein, M.D., of low-carbohydrate diet fame, never one to crumple in the face of conventional wisdom, has provided us with a dramatic incident that shows another side of the salt shaker. ▶**DiabetiLink #7**: A Pinch of Salt (See p. 272)

Le Flour du Mal

White flour is not as much of an active enemy as sugar and salt. Its fault lies not in what it does that's bad but rather in what it doesn't do that's good. The things that are taken out in the refining process are what's mainly good for you in the flour: the bran, which gives you fiber, and the wheat germ, which contains most of the nutrients (B vitamins, vitamin E, iron, and lysine).

Be ye not deceived by the word "enriched." This just means that some of the nutrients that were refined away have been restored. Almost all the trace elements—those appearing in minute quantities—are still gone and, of these, some—such as zinc and chromium—have been considered of special importance for diabetics.

One thing to remember if you decide to switch from white to whole-wheat flour is that whole-wheat flour is a perishable commodity. Try to buy it from a store where you know there's a rapid turnover and where they keep it in a cool place. When you get it home, keep it cool; we usually keep ours in the refrigerator. If you can find it, buy stone-ground whole-wheat flour, because fewer of the vitamins are destroyed than in the usual steel-roller milling, which raises the temperature of the wheat. Also, stone-ground flour stays fresher longer.

But since we all often buy our whole-wheat bread rather than baking it ourselves, what do you look for in that case? In packaged bread, look at the ingredients list and see if there is any coloring element lurking. Sometimes the whole wheat is more a matter of color rather than actuality. But truly you're better off eschewing the supermarket and going to a baker, where you can find whole *grain* bread, which is higher in fiber and vitamins and minerals. Particularly seek out the bakeries that make the increasingly available and popular artisan bread. If you ask what's the difference, you can find your answer on the website www.foodproductdesign.com in an article, "Simple

Steps to Artisan Breads" by Kirk O'Donnell, Ed.D., vice president of education at the American Institute of Baking.

What's the Difference?		
	WHITE PAN BREAD	**ARTISAN BREAD**
External apearance	Rectangular, uniform	Various Shapes
Crust	Thin	Thick
Texture	Soft	Chewy
Grain	Closed	Open
Shelf life	Long	Short

We might also mention that the artisan breads are often made with such ingredients as certified organic flour, filtered water, and pure sea salt, and that they have a heavenly aroma. We won't mention the difference in price, but we will say the artisan breads are worth every penny no matter how many pennies that may be.

For more information, search the Internet under the heading "Artisan Bread."

FRIEND OR FOE?

Milk, another white commodity, is not an enemy to most people, but it can be to some. While milk is generally known as the "perfect food" (especially by the dairy council!) and finds its way onto almost every kind of diabetes exchange list, it does have a few imperfections. For one thing, not everyone has the enzyme (lactase) to digest it. In fact, according to the *Harvard Medical School Health Letter,* 70 to 95 percent of persons of Mediterranean, black-African, and Asian ancestry lack it. Older people, too, sometimes have lost their milk-digesting enzyme. If someone without this enzyme is diagnosed as diabetic and conscientiously tries to consume the milk usually recommended on diabetic diets, it can cause digestive trouble that mimics an irritable colon condition: abdominal cramps, bloating, excessive gas, and diarrhea. If you suspect you may have this problem, your doctor can give you a test to determine if you have a lactase deficiency. People with a lactase deficiency can still enjoy the benefits of milk in such products as ripened cheeses and buttermilk because the lactose has, in effect, been predigested by bacterial cultures. They can also safely drink sweet acidophilus milk, which tastes just like regular milk. Best of all, now readily available in pharmacies are lactase enzyme replacement capsules such as Lactaid and Dairy Ease (many stores have their own generic brand). Using these opens new vistas of milk products that were previously forbidden to the lactose intolerant.

All diabetics should also remember that milk does contain a sugar—lactose. An eight-ounce glass gives you the equivalent of a half ounce of sugar, so it can raise your blood sugar. In fact, June uses it to treat hypoglycemia, as do many people in England. People on the low-carb diet who don't want that sugar can replace milk in recipes with half cream and half water. Of course you don't get the milk nutrients that way so you'll have to get your calcium, phosphorus, B_{12}, etc., from other food sources and supplements.

By all means, don't regard milk as an evil product, but do be alert to the disturbances that it can sometimes cause.

FAT CHANCE

As if you didn't have enough of them already, here's another dietary controversy for you to chew on. Is a high level of cholesterol in the bloodstream a risk factor for heart attack and stroke? And does your diet influence that cholesterol level?

Some studies indicate yes on both scores. For example, there was one made in Ethiopia, a country that has a low-fat, high-carbohydrate diet and that boasts a low heart-attack rate. The study was of 130 young-adult males—construction workers, college students, and bank employees—living in Addis Ababa. The construction workers ate the traditional diet, mainly whole-grain bread, vegetables, peas, and tea. Only on special occasions did they eat meat. The college students ate what the construction workers ate plus a little more fat from margarine and sausage. The bank clerks added butter, more meat, and a daily egg.

The results? The construction workers' cholesterol averaged 110 milligrams per 100 milliliters, the students averaged 160, and the bank clerks 180. (Young-adult male Americans average 200 and, at middle age, the average rises to 230. In countries where heart attacks are rare, the averages don't go over 200.)

Some scientists maintain that cholesterol studies like the preceding are still "inconclusive" and that since the body manufactures its own cholesterol anyway, what you eat isn't all that important. (Scientific studies are, of course, like the Bible. If you search long and hard enough you can usually find a quotation that justifies what you want to do.) We must admit, however, that in our opinion the weight falls on the side of those who *do* consider cholesterol a problem that can and should be avoided, and that changing your diet is the way to avoid it. Dr. Lawrence Power, writing in his syndicated "Food and Fitness" column, sums it up: "Many experts now regard a cholesterol of 200 as the upper limit of normal, a value that the average American exceeds in his twenties and can only reduce by cutting back on his fat-meat intakes and increasing his intake of vegetables and whole-grain foods like bread."

The 1986 report from the National Heart, Lung, and Blood Institute echoes these same sentiments. Their guidelines say that blood cholesterol should be below 200 milligrams and that in the 200 to 239 range a person is at moderate risk for coronary artery disease and at more than 240 at high risk. For those with cholesterol over 240, the institute recommends treatment first by diet and, if that fails, then by medication.

People at moderate or high risk should also have a test to determine the kinds of cholesterol in their blood. HDLs are high-density lipoproteins, the good guys, and LDLs are low-density lipoproteins, the bad guys. If you have very high HDLs they trump the LDLs. For example, June always has a cholesterol of over 200—sometimes as high as 230—but since her HDLs are so disproportionately high, she's in the low-risk category. That's why you shouldn't accept a general cholesterol number. Insist on getting HDL and LDL readings so you and your doctor can accurately evaluate your risk. Incidentally, the Eadeses, in their book *Protein Power,* have a different—and easier—way to figure your cholesterol. You divide the total cholesterol by your HDLs. To be out of the risk zone your total should be less than four. Then divide your LDL by your HDL. This result should be below three.

If you're tired of worrying about cholesterol, we offer for your masochistic pleasure another worrisome blood fat: triglycerides. The latest research shows that, like high cholesterol, high triglycerides increase heart-disease risk. They come from a combination of the fats and carbohydrates you eat. According to Jane Brody in her July 28, 1998, *New York Times* article on this subject:

> Diets high in saturated fats (from meat and dairy foods), sugars (including natural sugars in fruit), alcohol and refined carbohydrates (white bread, white rice, etc.) can raise blood levels of triglycerides. If people on a very low-fat diet replace fats with sugars and refined starches, triglyceride levels may rise and protective HDLs fall.

High blood sugars can also increase triglyceride levels—still another reason to keep your blood sugar normal!

The recommended triglyceride level used to be under 200, but this has been revised dramatically downward to under 100.

But no matter how you figure it, we believe that to be on the safe side—always the best side for a diabetic to be on—no matter which diet or combination of diets you follow, you should reduce the foods that tend to raise the level of fats and cholesterol and triglycerides in your bloodstream.

But on the other hand . . . ➤**DiabetiLink #8:** Extremism in the Reduction of Fat Is No Virtue (See p. 273)

The Unsaturation Point

In your personal fat-management program you should replace saturated fats as much as possible with unsaturated fats. It's fairly easy to recognize saturated fats, because they are usually solid or become solid when chilled. Saturated fats are the solid *animal* fats—the marbling that gives prime beef its flavor, the fat of bacon that crisps up so tastily when you fry it, butter, cheese, cream, the fat content in whole milk that gives it its richness, variety meats like sausage and salami, and solid cooking fats like lard.

They are also the vegetable fats coconut oil and palm oil. Although these vegetable fats do not *contain* cholesterol—no vegetable fat does—they do produce cholesterol in the body.

And there's a new Public Enemy on the risky fats scene: trans fat, which *Consumer Reports* labeled "The Stealth Fat" because it "lurks in a multitude of foods. It's not labeled. And it's bad for your heart." Studies indicate that trans fat increases the evil LDLs (the way saturated fats do), and here's the clincher: it decreases the good HDLs. Trans fat is what you get when polyunsaturated oil is partially hydrogenated so it can be made into margarine sticks that look like butter or into solid shortening used in many baked goods. The FDA is toying with the idea of requiring trans fats to be listed on food labels, but until that happens, you're pretty much on your own. A few labels now have the message "trans fatty acid–free." But if a product is *not* trans fatty acid–free, companies aren't likely to announce it on their packaging. One way, a way that requires some effort, is to add up the amount of saturated, monounsaturated, and polyunsaturated fats on the label and subtract that from the total fat. The remainder will be the trans fats. The good news is that food processors are being pressured to get rid of—or at least reduce the amount of—trans fat in their products, and many are starting to capitulate, including such big names as McDonald's and Frito Lay.

For more information on trans fat, including a list of products that contain trans fat, see the March 2003 issue of *Consumer Reports.*

Polyunsaturated fats are the liquid *vegetable* oils like corn, sesame, cottonseed, soybean, and safflower. Fish and poultry also contain more polyunsaturates than beef, lamb, and pork. They have always had favorable ratings.

But there have been recent reports indicating that monounsaturates are as good as or even better than polyunsaturates when it comes to preventing heart disease. One of the reasons for this theory comes from the fact that Italy and Greece—where olive oil, a 77-percent monounsaturate, is universally used—have the lowest rates of heart disease. Other high monounsaturates are canola, avocado, and macadamia-nut oils.

Currently our oils of choice are olive, avocado, and macadamia nut. Olive oils give a wonderful flavor to salads and sauces. June prefers the more delicate French olive oil, Barbara, the lustier Italian. In either case, since you don't use much of it, you should get the best, extra virgin (also called double virgin), which is from the first pressing of the olives. The second best is virgin, from the second pressing. We suggest avoiding the misnamed "pure" olive oil, which comes from treating the pressed-out olive pulp with chemicals, and the also misnamed "fine" olive oil, which is actually "pure" olive oil diluted with water.

Despite all of its virtues, olive oil has too pronounced a flavor for all kitchen uses. Avocado oil, we find, is ideal. This versatile oil is water-processed without chemicals or preservatives. It is 67 percent monounsaturates. It has a *very* high smoke point—over 300cc. This means that on those rare occasions when you fry foods, you can get the oil extremely hot before adding the foods; thus less oil is absorbed into the food. Avocado oil also has only 8.2 calories per gram rather than the 9 calories of most other oils and butter. You can reduce calories and cholesterol in recipes calling for butter by substituting one-half or even two-thirds of the butter with avocado oil. The flavor will still be there because avocado oil has something of a buttery taste itself. Incidentally, it doesn't taste at all like avocados, so even people who don't like avocados will enjoy it. It's also a great little emulsifier so you can easily whip up nice thick salad dressings and mayonnaise with it. Its only drawbacks were its expense and the fact that it was hard to find. But things are getting better. Starting in 2002, it began being distributed in the United States with more major chains—particularly the upscale ones—signing up every day. As it gets wider distribution and sales, the price is likely to creep in a downward direction. To find out where avocado oil is available in your part of the country contact Vicky M. Mathiesen, Natural Imports, phone: 949-442-8853; fax: 949-442-8811; e-mail: vmathiesen@att.net.

Macadamia nut oil is much easier to locate than avocado. But if you have trouble finding it in your local markets, there are several websites that offer it. Just enter "macadamia nut oil" on your search engine and there it is and there you are. It is 80 percent monounsaturates as compared to olive oil's 74 percent, and avocado oil's 67 percent. It has an even higher smoke point than avocado oil—389cc versus 300cc. It does have a pronounced flavor, albeit a delicious one, but if you want a purer taste, avocado would be a better bet.

WHERE CHOLESTEROL LURKS

Egg yolks are very high in cholesterol (one large egg yolk contains 252 milligrams). June's doctor hasn't had an egg in twelve years and his cholesterol is 150. But just to keep the controversy alive, we ought to tell you that there are those who say eggs contain lecithin, which negates their cholesterol (sigh!). When it comes to eggs, what we generally do is leave half the yolks out in scrambled eggs or omelettes and in most recipes calling for eggs. (This usually means adding extra eggs, because if you're using fewer yolks you need more whites.) There are also a number of egg substitutes on the market. If you decide to use these, Dr. Anderson suggests you select the ones with fewer than 200 calories per cup.

Organ meats such as liver and kidney are extremely high in cholesterol. If you're a liver fancier and feel that giving it up would be a great loss, remember that the liver in animals is a great depository of DDT and other noxious chemicals that might be even more disastrous to your health than cholesterol. If you give up liver and other organ meats, you'll be avoiding these poisons as well as cholesterol.

Shellfish are on the high-cholesterol list, alas! But the recent scientific position is that even though shellfish are relatively high in cholesterol, they're so low in saturated fat that even if you're on a low-cholesterol diet you don't have to eliminate them entirely. Oysters, clams, and scallops are the lowest in cholesterol and are the preferred choice. Shrimp, lobster, and crab, although higher in cholesterol, are again, low in saturated fat, so with them, too, you're okay; but watch the amounts you eat more closely.

We're always on the lookout for new saturated fat- and cholesterol-avoidance ideas. And, of course, we are not alone. Manufacturers have long been working in their labs to develop a fat substitute, literally a nonfat fat. Two such substances are now being used in commercial products: NutraSweet's Simplesse and Procter & Gamble's Olestra. Simplesse is a low-fat fat not suitable for cooking. It is composed of whey protein from milk or egg whites (beware if you have an allergy to either) and replaces 27 calories of fat with 4 calories of protein. Olestra is mainly sucrose and vegetable oil bonded into molecules too large to digest. It can be used in cooking.

An Olestrsa negative that has been reported in studies is that it removes fat-soluble vitamins from the body and reduces beta-carotene levels. Simplesse, too, is said to interfere with the absorption of important nutrients. Taste is also a factor to consider. They just don't have the same flavor as regular fats.

So stay on your guard with these and other dietary miracles that come onto the market. Use your own ingenuity in playing the low-fat game. It's a challenge and, in its own way, fun—something like doing the *New York Times* crossword puzzle. If you get into the spirit of it, you'll soon develop your own set of tricks to eliminate saturated fats and cholesterol and the alleged cardiovascular problems that go along with them, and still enjoy your meals.

Control through Control

And here's a final tip on controlling your cholesterol. One of the best ways to do it is through keeping your diabetes in good control. According to Dr. Julio Rosenstock of the University of Texas Health Science Center, doing so will "lower a patient's plasma cholesterol, low-density lipoprotein cholesterol [the bad cholesterol], and triglyceride levels."

VEGETARIANISM

Vegetarianism, or at least cutting back on red meat in the diet, is becoming a way of eating for people with all kinds of health problems, as well as for those who have no health problems and want to keep it that way. Many young people are adopting vegetarianism as an act of conscience or, some say, as an act of defiance and hostility toward their parents! If, for whatever reason, you lean toward a vegetarian diet, your diabetes won't prevent you from following that inclination. Whether you follow the standard Exchange List diet, the HCF diet, or variations thereon, you should have no problem being a vegetarian although you will have to take certain precautions and make certain adjustments. If you want to follow the low-carb diet, you must have already figured out that you can't be a vegetarian on it. You'll have to choose whichever one is more important to you.

If you want to be a lacto-ovo vegetarian on the HCF diet, you'll have to make it nonfat lacto-egg-white (or egg substitute). To be a vegan (one who consumes neither eggs or milk products nor meat, poultry, or fish) on HCF would be a natural. With the standard diabetes diet, you could be a lacto-ovo or, with a great deal of tightrope walking, a vegan.

If you want to adopt either kind of vegetarian diet, you have to study and learn a great deal. Fortunately, there are excellent books to refer to. Marion Franz, R.D., in *Exchanges for All Occasions,* has an entire chapter called "If You Want to Be a Vegetarian," in which she provides a list of special vegetarian exchanges.

We also heartily recommend *The New Laurel's Kitchen.* Its philosophy is beautiful, the recipes delicious and totally unlike some of the strange ersatz guck sometimes served up in the name of vegetarianism, and the scientific dietary information is impeccable and understandable. *The New Laurel's Kitchen,* again unlike many vegetarian cookbooks, is against the use of excessive amounts of sweets and fats, which makes it especially good for diabetics. We also recommend and use ourselves *Complete Vegetarian Cooking,* edited by Sunset Books and Sunset Magazine (this includes a nutritional analysis of each recipe), *The Vegetarian Epicure: Book Two* by Anna Thomas (her *New Vegetarian Epicure* talks turkey—literally and shows how to carve one!), and *Greene on Greens.* Two vegetarian books aimed especially toward people with diabetes are *Beyond Alfalfa Sprouts and Cheese* by Judy Gilliard and Joy Kirkpatrick, R.D. (now out-of-print, but available used on the Internet from Amazon.com and half.com) and *Vegetarian Cooking for People with Diabetes* by Patricia Le Shane.

As more and more people become interested in vegetarianism, whether for moral, health, or economic reasons, more and more good vegetarian cookbooks are bound to appear. Watch for them, and especially for ones written for diabetics.

SOY TO THE WORLD

It would seem that there is finally something that is considered the ideal food for everyone—soy. It's beginning to look as if this inexpensive, ubiquitous food known for almost three thousand years should be a staple in everyone's diet.

This multifaceted legume contains a healthy balance of proteins, carbohydrates, fat, vitamins, minerals, and fiber. It's cholesterol-free, lactose-free, and low in saturated fat. An analysis of a 3.2 ounce serving of one form of soy, tofu (bean curd), is: 90 calories, 11 grams of protein, 1 gram of carbohydrate, and 5 grams of fat. Soy is distinctive and valuable because it is mainly protein. Here is the solution to your protein quandary if you want to cut back on the animal fat varieties.

Dr. James Anderson, the father of the HCF diet, the oat bran hero of the 1970s, and the author of *Diabetes: A Practical New Guide to Healthy Living,* has been researching the health-protecting aspects of soy. He reports his findings in his new book, *Dr. Anderson's Antioxidant, Antiaging Health Program.* Apparently he's convinced himself of the merits of soy because he's now consuming a minimum of 18 grams of soy protein daily and some days 33 to 38 grams. He's this committed to soy protein because he has learned that it:

- Reduces the risk of cancer, heart disease, and osteoporosis
- Lowers blood cholesterol and triglyceride levels
- Protects against kidney disease in diabetics
- May reduce adverse symptoms of menopause

In what form can you find this beneficent bean? There is tofu (soybean curd), soy yogurt, soy flour, soy milk, soy nuts, and even tempeh, an Indonesian soy cake. Many of us eat about half a cup of soybeans every day without realizing it, because they're found in nondairy creamers, mayonnaise, shortening, bread, soups, oils, etc. There are over 400 soy products on the market in the United States today. In fact two-thirds of the world's soybean crop is grown in this country. Barbara has become a believer in starting the day the low-carb, high-protein way with a glass of soymilk enhanced with a teaspoon of vanilla and a half-package of non-calorie sweetener and accompanied by a muffin made from one of Atkins' Kitchen Quick and Easy Muffin mixes. (Her favorite is corn.)

We became so enthralled with soy that we attended the Tofu Festival in Los Angeles's Little Tokyo area. Twenty-six restaurants served a tasty variety of tofu dishes ranging from miso soup and tofu curry to more far-out peanut butter tofu and tofu chocolate mousse and tofu cheesecake. We shared a tofu Caesar salad and shrimp and cheese tofu balls.

Since it's unlikely that you'll make it to the next Tofu Festival, to give you an idea of how versatile and interesting tofu can be, here's a recipe from Fran McCullough's wonderful cookbook, *Living Low Carb.*

SCRAMBLED TOFU

Sometimes the idea of more eggs for breakfast is just unappealing but you can't think of anything else. Tofu is lighter and has a nice texture. If you want an eggy yellow look, add a pinch of turmeric.

1 tablespoon olive oil
2 scallions, minced, including
    some of the green
10-ounce box silken tofu, drained
Big pinch of turmeric
    (optional)

Salt and pepper
Hot pepper sauce
½ cup grated cheddar or jack
    cheese (optional)
Paprika

Heat the oil in a skillet and sauté the scallions until they're soft, about 3 minutes. Meanwhile, crumble the tofu. Stir the tofu into the pan with the turmeric, if you're using it. Add salt, pepper, and hot pepper sauce to taste. Cook over high heat until the tofu is firm, about 2 to 3 minutes.

Add the optional cheese and sprinkle with paprika. Serve hot. Serves 2.

PER SERVING   CARBOHYDRATE: 4.5 gm plus 0.8 gm fiber
PROTEIN: 10.2 gm   FAT: 10.6 gm

Incidentally, Fran's other cookbook, *The Low Carb Cookbook,* is equally outstanding and includes three other recipes for tofu plus tofu tips. P.S. You don't have to be on the low-carb diet to use Fran's recipes, you just have to enjoy good food.

From all this good news about the merits of soy, you'd think it has no flaws whatsoever. But some dietary someone somewhere somehow can always come up with something wrong. ➤**DiabetiLink #9:** No Joy in Soyville (See p. 274)

GARLIC: THE SCENTIMENTAL FAVORITE

In olden times in certain cultures children were trundled off to school wearing a bag filled with garlic cloves to ward off the seasonal diseases.

It worked, probably because the odoriferous garlic served to keep germ carriers at bay. But the haunting aroma is about the only negative we can think of for what is sometimes called the wonder herb.

Here are some of the many benefits this benevolent bulb is said to bestow upon those who partake of it (you will note that many of these relate to conditions to which people with diabetes are susceptible):

1. It lowers cholesterol and triglycerides. Who says? Steven Warshafsky at the New York Medical College, Valhalla, in reviewing garlic and cholesterol studies, found that people with cholesterol in excess of 200 were able to lower their levels by about 9 percent through the use of one-half to one clove of garlic a day. In a study in Germany, 261 patients were given either garlic powder tablets or a placebo. Within twelve weeks of this treatment, cholesterol dropped by 12 percent in the group taking garlic and the triglycerides went down 17 percent. The levels of the placebo-takers remained the same.

2. It keeps LDL cholesterol from oxidizing, which in turn keeps the plaque from building up on artery walls, which, again in turn, reduces heart attack and stroke risk. Who says? University of Kansas researchers who found that taking 600 milligrams of powdered garlic every day for two weeks lowered LDL oxidation by 34 percent.

3. It kills bacteria and viruses. Who says? Early on, Louis Pasteur pronounced it an effective antibiotic. In 1944, chemist Chester J. Cavallito discovered that allicin (a substance found in garlic) had antibiotic powers as effective as those in penicillin or tetracycline, and James North, a microbiologist at Brigham Young University, discovered in tests that it kills cold and flu viruses. ("Take two cloves of garlic, go to bed, and call me in the morning.") Note: According to the Garlic Information Center, "It is known that the most sensitive bacterium to garlic is the deadly *Bacillus anthracis,* which produces the poison anthrax."

4. It lowers blood pressure. Who says? Dr. F. G. Piotrowski of the University of Geneva tested garlic on one hundred patients. Forty percent of these had a drop of 20 millimeters in blood pressure in only one week. It is his theory that garlic inflates blood vessels, thereby reducing blood pressure. His patients' symptoms of dizziness, anginalike pain, and headaches diminished five days after the start of the experiment. Garlic has been used for blood-pressure lowering in China for centuries. Fifty bazillion Chinese can't be wrong!

Want some more benefits of garlic? Okay. It's as effective or better than aspirin as a blood thinner and anticoagulant, it helps fight herpes and skin lesions such as warts, and studies are beginning to indicate that it may help people avoid breast, liver, and colon cancer. Is it any wonder that the ancient Egyptians worshiped it?

How should you take your garlic? There are garlic pills (one way to avoid the breath that drives vampires away) but it's more beneficial (and enjoyable!) to eat it in food. We're of the opinion that many of the health benefits of the Mediterranean diet attributed to olive oil really belong to garlic—or garlic should at least be credited with an assist.

The most effective way of all is to eat garlic raw. Some determined garlic True Believers chop it up in little pieces and swallow it like pills. Daily. But why do that when there are many delicious dishes that use garlic in its natural state. One of these is aïoli—pronounced I-oh-lee (with the accent on the lee).

Aïoli

In summer in the south of France, many communities stage a "Grand Aïoli" sometimes even called a "Monstre Aïoli." This is a big party to bring together the citizens of the town and any lucky tourists who happen to be passing through. One summer when we were visiting friends in Ménerbes, a picturesque town deep in the heart of Peter Mayle country they had a Grand Aïoli complete with music and wine and all manner of food—cod, snails, artichokes, cauliflower, leeks, fennel, haricots verts (French green beans), hard-boiled eggs, crusty French bread, many varieties of local olives, and just about anything else they could think of at the time. The heart of the matter, though, is the aïoli, which you could call a garlicky mayonnaise, but if you called it that it would be a gross understatement of its merits. There are as many aïoli recipes as there are cooks in Provence, but here is one from the now out-of-print *The Flavor of France* by the photographer Samuel Chamberlain and his French wife, Narcisse. We're particularly fond of it since it is both authentic and easy to prepare.

AÏOLI PROVENÇAL

Use as many cloves of garlic in the aïoli as you dare. The correct recipe calls for 8 cloves per cup of homemade mayonnaise: 3 cloves is about the minimum if the dish is to keep its character. Start with the garlic, minced and mashed to a pulp, in a bowl. With a sauce whisk beat in 2 egg yolks. Add ¼ teaspoon of salt and a little freshly ground pepper; then add, drop by drop, 4 tablespoons of chilled olive oil, stirring furiously. Pour this mixture into an electric blender, turn the blender on and slowly add the juice of ½ lemon and 1 tablespoon of lukewarm water. Then gradually add 1 cup of chilled olive oil. Do not make more than one cup of aïoli at a time in an electric blender.

True confession: In a pinch we've been known to make aïoli with commercial mayonnaise, adding a touch of olive oil for flavor. But we try to stay out of a pinch.

By the way, if you're afraid of offending friends with your garlic miasma, we offer the solution of one of our friends. She refuses to have any friends that don't like and consume garlic. We are happy to still be included among her friends.

THE FRUIT, THE WHOLE FRUIT, AND NOTHING BUT THE FRUIT

Over the years June has given up drinking fruit juice in any circumstances except to counteract insulin reactions. She found that the juice shot her blood sugar up in a way that the fruit itself didn't seem to. This discovery was later confirmed by Dr. Lawrence Power in his *Food and Fitness* newspaper column: "Fruit juice can give your system a jolt. . . . Recent studies by nutrition scientists reveal that a six-ounce glass of any natural fruit juice will sharply increase blood-sugar levels to a peak." In nondiabetics, he explained, this can cause the body to overreact, sending out insulin resulting in hypoglycemia with its old familiar episodes of shaking, sweating, and anxiety. We all know what a sugar jolt like that does to a diabetic.

This blood-sugar peaking rarely occurs after eating the whole fruit; apparently the pulp slows down the action. We've also noticed that for snacks on the HCF diet, Dr. Anderson recommends a piece of whole-wheat bread or some rye crackers in conjunction with fresh fruit. The fiber of the bread exchange slows the fruit down even further.

Incidentally, if you're in the habit of drinking orange juice made from a frozen concentrate, you might be interested in Dr. Power's description of that product: "Frozen orange juice is really a concentrate of sugar from the orange. . . . Oranges by the truckload are dumped on a conveyer belt, scrubbed clean, split and reamed, and the juice filtered to remove pulp (and thus any nutrient contribution the pulp might make) and seeds. It then enters a holding tank, where it is heated to kill any germs, and vacuum-evaporated to a thick, orange-colored sugar syrup." And that's what you defrost, dilute, and drink.

VITAMINS AND MINERALS AND HERBS

Supplements

We always wear kid gloves when entering the vitamin/mineral supplement arena. No health subject is more fraught with controversy and contradiction. Dr. Ron Brown, our old friend and employee when we had the SugarFree Center, is a triple-threat man: R.D., M.D., *and* he has type 1 diabetes. He offers what we have come to think is the soundest advice. If you have no known vitamin deficiencies, your best bet is to get all your vitamins and minerals from your good-and-healthy balanced meal plan. But just as a safety net, Ron advises one multivitamin tablet a day.

This kind of uniform one-a-day prescription does not, of course, apply to all people of all ages and sexes. Women, in particular, usually need extra calcium and/or iron. The recommended daily dietary allowance (RDA) of calcium for women is 800 to 1,000 milligrams, but growing girls and pregnant and lactating women need at least 1,200 to 1,400 milligrams a day. (A glass of milk usually contains 300 milligrams of calcium.) Postmenopausal women not receiving estrogen should have at least 1,500 milligrams daily. (To get that amount, you'd need the equivalent of two quarts of milk.) As you can see, what supplements to take and the amounts is another of those manifold check-with-your-doctor activities.

In spite of our cautious attitude, we want to make you aware that new studies are showing that some diabetics (particularly those who are out of control and producing excess urine) may suffer from vitamin C deficiency, and supplements of 1,500 milligrams a day may improve their A1c tests. Vitamin E (400 to 800 international units) may do the same thing. These two vitamins (antioxidants) are also thought to protect against heart disease and cancer. ➤**DiabetiLink #10: Oh Say Should You C?** (See p. 275)

Two trace minerals—zinc and chromium—have been touted by many of the antiestablishment diet and health books and magazines as having blood-sugar–lowering benefits for diabetics. The scientific evidence on which these claims are based has to do with the following facts: zinc plays a role in carbohydrate metabolism, chromium deficiency can raise blood glucose, and chromium supplementation improves glucose tolerance in some older people. However, we can find no large-scale studies that give conclusive results on these two minerals for diabetics. The consensus is that taking supplements of these will help if you have a deficiency. Otherwise they won't make any difference and are unnecessary. We therefore favor waiting for definitive evidence of their benefits before loading up on these supplements. (If you do read of studies showing supplements of either of these do great things for all people with diabetes, consider the source. If the studies were done under the auspices of a company producing or selling the mineral, that should activate your skepticism gland.)

Another supplement craze has been fish oil, in particular the omega-3 fatty acids found in cold-water fish like salmon, herring, sardines, mackerel, tuna, cod, shrimp, lobster, crab, and the like. Researchers found that omega-3s lowered cholesterol and triglycerides and removed some of the risk of heart attack and stroke. More recently, however, warnings have come out about the possible dangers of high-dosage supplements of omega-3. In fact, they are not recommended by the American Diabetes Association or the American Heart Association, and the latest indication that they can be dangerous is that the FDA has ordered manufacturers to stop further distribution. The best advice we can give you is to eat cold-water fish at least twice a week for your omega-3s. But you should be doing that anyway: fish is a very healthy food.

Herbs

One day, back in our SugarFree Center days, a gentleman came in and asked, "Say, what do you people do here?" "We try to help people with diabetes take good care of themselves," we answered.

He lowered his voice conspiratorially, "You know they don't *have* to have diabetes. We can get rid of it for them." He gestured to a newly opened store across the street. It displayed a banner with the name of a well-known herbal supplement. We were relieved when the store closed down in a few months because their stock-in-trade was false hope and misinformation and who-knows-what potentially damaging herbal products.

This is not to malign all herbs as specious and dangerous. Some, such as our beloved garlic, and other commonly used kitchen herbs and spices like cinnamon, ginger, and sage, and the lesser-known fenugreek, have been proven beneficial—and non-deleterious—down through the ages. Nevertheless, many herbs, along with certain vitamins and minerals, remain controversial and confusing. To try to clear up the muddy waters on those topics, we've called in an expert, Diana W. Guthrie, Ph.D., FAAN, CDE, BC-ADM. She is a retired professor at the University of Kansas School of Medicine, trained in both traditional and nontraditional care, and is a recipient of the American Diabetes Association's Outstanding Educator Award. Her recent book, *Alternative and Complementary Diabetes Care: How to Combine Natural and Traditional Therapies,* is uniquely valuable for those who want to explore other avenues to improved diabetes control. We asked Dr. Guthrie to give us a selection of "Picks," vitamins, minerals, and herbs that could be of value to people with diabetes and "Nix" those that are overrated and/or dangerous.

Diana W. Guthrie's Picks

Alpha lipoic acid is getting a good track record in treating and/or preventing mild polyneuropathy.

Bilberry has been found to have some effect on diabetes. The leaves are the part that have been found useful in lowering blood glucose levels in people with type 2 diabetes. Bilberry is also known by the names of *arandano* in Spain, blueberry in Europe, and whortleberry. Watch out for the raw berries, as they can aggravate diarrhea.

B-complex is helpful when the person is in a stressed state. It is believed to work on the nerves and as a sedative. It may be found in chickweed. The constituents include B_1, B_2, B_6, B_{12}, biotin, chrome, folic acid, pantothenic acid, and B_3 (niacin). Niacin raises blood sugar but lowers cholesterol, except that the extended-release niacin does not appear to raise blood sugar. It has a side effect of flushing of the face and sometimes nausea. Niacin breaks down into nicotinamide, which affects the blood glucose levels by enhancing the work of the pancreas and protecting the beta cells. It does not appear to raise blood glucose levels, and in Australia and Europe has been used in studies, many with children, to possibly prevent progression on to insulin-dependent diabetes (type 1).

Bitter Melon might prove to be useful, if it is offered as a standardized product. In a study it did lower blood sugar 25 percent when ingested over a three-week period.

COQ_{10} is thought to assist the immune system and act as an antioxidant. It is also useful for reducing side effects when having chemotherapy. There is some word on its effect on blood sugars, but as yet there are no strong studies indicating this.

Cinnamon, used medicinally in China since 2700 B.C. has antiseptic qualities. For diabetes, cinnamon has been shown by the U.S. Department of Agriculture researchers to aid insulin and its association in glucose metabolism. But so far, dosages have not been studied to the point of usefulness in relation to diabetes treatment.

Ginger is said to aid with stomach upset. Some say that it prevents motion sickness when taken half an hour before a trip. This could be helpful for people with diabetes, since nausea and vomiting could lead to hypoglycemia.

Fenugreek seeds are high in fiber and have been shown to aid in reducing blood sugar, as noted by studies carried out in India. It is now available under the label of Limitrol. Limitrol is a new way to limit glucose absorption naturally. It also limits fat and calorie absorption.

Ginseng is a blend of Pix and Nix. This two-thousand-year-old remedy is reported to increase energy, elevate moods, reduce fasting blood sugars, improve work performance, and even act as a mild aphrodisiac. It is possible that the increased energy and elevated mood may cause the person to become more active and burn more calories, thereby lowering blood sugars. On the Nix side, side effects have linked ginseng to insomnia, diarrhea, vaginal bleeding, and painful breasts. Ginseng becomes less effective when taken continually and should not be taken for more than two to three weeks at a time, tops, with a week or so break before restarting.

Milk thistle is helpful for those who have "injured" livers, changes from medications, etc.

Diana W. Guthrie's Nixes

Human Growth Hormone is a no-no. It relates indirectly with elevated blood-glucose levels and can be quite harmful to the body. It has been used by sports enthusiasts to build up muscle bulk. It is known for leading to cardiovascular problems.

Stay away from *Ma Huang* (ephedra). Already damaged blood vessels may be broken with the increased blood pressure associated with this herb. It is dangerous when used without professional guidance.

Yohimbine has been used in the treatment of physiologically based erectile dysfunction, but it is one of those herbs that can have dangerous side effects. This must be administered by a qualified person. There are also a number of other herbs that have been used to treat erectile dysfunction, but either they are even less effective or they have greater side effects.

Diana W. Guthrie's General Cautions

If it sounds too good to be true, it probably is.

Natural does not necessarily mean safe.

More is not better unless supported by research.

Only try and, if desired to do so, add one herb at a time. That way there is less chance of getting confused as to what is experienced and its relationship to the herb.

CHEMICALS

June became very conscious of chemicals in foods during her headache years because many chemicals, notably MSG and nitrates or nitrites, were known to cause headaches. Since a headache is a common symptom of low blood sugar, a diabetic who doesn't want to have to deal with confusing body signals would naturally want to avoid headache-producing substances. On top of that, these chemicals have other side effects that are detrimental to your health.

Take the "flavor enhancer" MSG—or, rather, *don't* take it if you can avoid it. When you read labels you'll find it's in almost every processed food. Besides producing headaches in susceptible individuals, it also produces dizziness, nasal congestion, and general feelings of malaise, among others. But that's not the worst of it. MSG is monosodium glutamate. That sodium is the same old sodium that does you wrong in salt, and it does you wrong in exactly the same ways.

Nitrates and nitrites are suspected cancer producers, and cancer does not improve diabetes. Actually, you have a double reason for avoiding nitrates and nitrites. They are usually found in things like bacon, sausage, hot dogs, and lunch meats, which are also full of another item high on the diabetes nix list: fat.

Besides these known enemy chemicals in food, there are hundreds of unknowns that are currently on the Federal Drug Administration's GRAS (Generally Regarded as Safe) list. Remember, though, a goodly number of the chemicals that are now forbidden in food were once "generally regarded as safe" by the FDA. A chemical is like an accused person in our system of justice: innocent until proven guilty. To be on the safe side, we prefer to shun as many of these potential criminals as possible. This usually means reading the label, rejecting the product, sighing heavily, and deciding to fix the food from scratch, using fresh ingredients.

Unfortunately, even fresh ingredients are suspect these days, what with the wide use of chemical fertilizers and pesticides. Health-food stores advertise their vegetables, fruits, and grains as "organically grown" and claim that they are free from all harmful chemicals. We've read several studies, however, showing that these fruits and vegetables often come from the same bins in the very same whole-sale-produce markets as those you find in the supermarket. The only thing that's different about them is the higher price. That's why we shop mostly at farmer's markets.

One important change is the Nutrition Labeling and Education Act of 1990, mandating easier-to-understand nutrition labels on most prepared foods by May 1993. The FDA must also define those ambiguous terms *natural, fresh,* and *organic,* which have been used for years to trick us into purchasing items that, if the truth be known, we would rather not consume. We must pray now that these admirable intentions will not be thwarted by special interests pressuring the Department of Agriculture.

CAFFEINE

Diabetic dietitian Meg Gaekle calls coffee "the last vestige of diabetic freedom." So it is! This nice, comforting beverage is a mood elevator well known for its ability literally to wake you up and make you more alert. It has now even been scientifically substantiated that coffee decreases fatigue and makes you think more clearly. No wonder we naturally gravitate toward it.

So what's wrong with drinking coffee? The psychoactive drug in coffee is, of course, caffeine. And over the years we've all heard that caffeine does terrible things to your body. It's been accused of causing heart disease, high blood pressure, high blood-cholesterol levels, and different forms of cancer, including pancreatic—all the things diabetics in particular don't need.

But now, thanks to large-scale scientific studies by qualified researchers, caffeine is losing its evil image. It's now being reported that you're safe from those reputed damaging physical effects if you keep your consumption of caffeine to no more than two or three cups a day. This is certainly welcome news, because coffee is *free* in the diabetic sense of the word. And, of course, so is tea, which also contains caffeine. So are sugar-free soft drinks, many of which also contain caffeine. The following chart from the FDA shows the caffeine content of a five-ounce serving of hot beverages and a twelve-ounce serving of soft drinks, as well as other sources of caffeine. Two hundred milligrams of caffeine a day appear to be a safe amount for most people (those with heart arrhythmias are an exception).

Decaffeinated coffee: 2–5 mg	Instant tea: 25–50 mg
Percolated coffee: 40–170 mg	Cocoa: 2–20 mg
Drip-brewed coffee: 60–185 mg	Many soft drinks: 30–55 mg
Instant coffee: 30–120 mg	Weight-loss drugs, diuretics: 100–200 mg
Brewed tea: 20–115 mg	Pain relievers: 30–100 mg
Cold/allergy remedies: 15–30 mg	

What if you overdo on caffeine? It can make you very nervous and jumpy as well as create a bad case of insomnia. And the amount of coffee that you can drink without experiencing adverse symptoms is a very individual matter. Much depends on whether you're a regular consumer. If you regularly drink 250 milligrams a day (two to three cups), caffeine will have no significant effect on your blood pressure, heart rate, respiration, metabolic rate, blood-glucose concentration, or cholesterol level. But if you haven't had any for a week or two, the effects may be more pronounced.

Speaking of blood-glucose levels, coffee does cause blood sugar to rise somewhat. It also aggravates ulcers, and, most seriously, it does "hasten the excretion of calcium from the body, which could increase the risk of osteoporosis," according to the *Johns Hopkins Medical Letter* of March 1991. Another negative: since caffeine is a drug, it has withdrawal symptoms, mainly headache and fatigue. It takes about a week to lose these symptoms (don't take a caffeine-containing over-the-counter painkiller when giving up caffeine!).

Giving Coffee a Break

Because of dire reports of coffee's ill-effects, guilt has often tempered our enjoyment of this aromatic beverage, but good news is starting to filter out about it. A *Reader's Digest* article discussed a Danish study that showed how caffeine may have a role in weight control because it raises the rate at which the body burns calories. Just 100 milligrams of caffeine (about one cup of coffee) can raise the metabolism rate at least 3 to 4 percent. And the caloric burn stimulated by caffeine is even greater when combined with exercise. What's more, a Canadian study says caffeine helps make body fat available as a fuel for exercising muscles so that they work longer before they fatigue.

And *New York Times* health writer Jane Brody reports that, contrary to the current belief that women who drink too much coffee will have bone loss and an increased risk of osteoporosis, a new study at the Hershey Medical Center in Pennsylvania produced a strong "maybe not" on the subject. No relationship was found between women's bone density whether they drank zero to two cups, three to four cups, or five or more cups of coffee with caffeine a day.

Here's yet another positive report. Chemicals in coffee (both caffeinated and decaffeinated) may form potent antioxidants similar to vitamin C or vitamin E, which are believed to help prevent cancer. Dr. Takayuki Shibamoto, a University of California at Davis professor of environmental toxicology, reports that his preliminary study indicates "the antioxidants in a cup of coffee might be equal to the amount found in three oranges." The only caveat is that you have to drink your coffee in about twenty minutes after it is brewed to benefit from the antioxidants.

All that good news should perk up coffee lovers everywhere.

Our compromise with coffee drinking, in view of all this new research, is to grind together half regular and half decaffeinated beans.

Your Health Is in the Bag (Tea, That Is)

When it comes to caffeine, Americans primarily get their fixes in coffee and cola, whereas the British, Chinese, Japanese, and East Indians all go for tea. It's come to light that maybe that's why their heart disease rates are so much lower than ours, especially among the green tea drinkers of the Far East. We remember that when we were visiting some of the World War II battlefields in the Netherlands we were told that the British army would put down their arms every afternoon and brew themselves a nice cup of tea right on the battlefield. It turns out that's not as crazy as we thought.

According to a London study, "One cup of tea a day could cut risk of heart attack by 44 percent." Tea contains flavonoids, which are powerful antioxidants. Antioxidants prevent cell damage and protect against heart disease and cancer.

Jane Brody of the *New York Times* went even further in praising the benefits of tea—green, black, and oolong. Green tea, she reports, is the least processed and therefore the healthiest. It has as much caffeine as black tea (about 40 milligrams per cup versus drip coffee, which has at least 100 milligrams per cup.) Instant teas don't have many protective chemicals.

The evidence favoring the health-giving properties of green and black tea have caused the National Cancer Institute to initiate studies to ascertain the capacity of the chemical in these teas to curb the development of cancer in people at high risk for cancers of the colon, lungs, esophagus, and skin.

Dr. James Anderson, in his latest book, *Dr. Anderson's Antioxidant, Antiaging Health Program,* recommends two cups of green or black tea daily. We're happy to say that June, who is one-quarter English, always demands an afternoon tea break British style, with a little cream. (Her genes make her do it!) We use Yorkshire Gold bags imported from England.

But if you feel that caffeine in any beverage affects you adversely, there is always the alternative of herbal teas, although these are not always harmless. Some ginseng teas have up to 85 percent sugar, and this may not be on the label. Above all, don't let anyone tell you that you can cure diabetes with any kind of herbal tea.

FALLING IN LOVE WITH CHOCOLATE

If you love chocolate, there's a good reason why. Scientists have discovered that eating chocolate produces the same chemical in the brain (phenylethylamine) as falling in love, thereby producing feelings of euphoria. That's why, when love has gone, people often go on chocolate binges to try to recapture that certain feeling.

There's more reason than that to turn to chocolate, as *USA Today* reported in their International edition of September 23, 1996: Doctors advise having a piece of chocolate along with a glass of red wine because they're both good and good for you, Researchers at the University of California at Davis, where they have an oenology course and are therefore interested in wine, say both wine and chocolate contain phenols, chemicals believed to help stop arteries from clogging up. "The pleasant pairing of red wine and dark chocolate," they say, "could have synergistic advantages beyond their complimentary taste." It's significant for people with diabetes that the recommendation is for *dark* chocolate. It has fewer calories and carbohydrates than milk chocolate and, according to a Valentine's Day column by Jane Brody in the *New York Times,* it does not promote tooth decay. Dark chocolate is also a more elegant and refined product. Stanley Marcus, the late chairman of Neiman Marcus, refused to allow milk chocolate in his stores, saying "Milk chocolate is a rube taste."

There has also been a recent claim that there is a link between chocolate and marijuana in the sense that chocolate gives you the same kind of high. All we can say is that if you eat too much chocolate, you may get an unwelcome high—high blood sugar.

The belief is that chocolate is high in caffeine and shouldn't be eaten before going to bed. Not so. Chocolate does have some caffeine, but not much. An ounce of dark (there we go again!) chocolate contains a mere 5 to 10 milligrams of caffeine, whereas a five- to six-ounce cup of coffee contains 100 to 150 milligrams.

Although chocolate is high in fat—that's what gives it such a great "mouth feel"—much of the fat in chocolate is made up of stearic acid, which does not raise blood cholesterol as much as other types of saturated fat.

So in moderation you can feel safe following the advice of an Internet philosopher: "Put 'eat chocolate' at the top of your list of things to do today. That way, at least you'll get one thing done."

ONE FOR THE ROAD; TO DRINK OR NOT TO DRINK

(Note: If you are religiously or morally or for any other personal reason opposed to drinking, you don't need to read this section. Just stay the way you are.) We once heard a wise dietitian speaking at a diabetes seminar. She told her fellow dietitians that when a diabetic patient asks if it's all right to have a cocktail before dinner or a glass or two of wine with dinner, it's not much help to say, "You'll have to ask your doctor about that." It's not much help, she said, because we all know full well what the doctor will say. The doctor who's a teetotaler will say, "Absolutely not. No alcohol at all. Not a drop." The doctor who's *not* a teetotaler will say, "I don't think a cocktail or a glass of wine will hurt you."

So what is a diabetic supposed to do when it comes to drinking? We suggest looking at the facts and making an intelligent decision based on your own lifestyle. Actually, that's what we suggest in all areas of diabetes care.

There are many reasons not to drink:

- Alcoholic drinks contain calories and, in some cases, carbohydrates.
- If weight is a problem for you, drinking can augment that problem. If you do drink, you have to count the alcohol as part of your diet. If you're already on a low-calorie diet to lose weight and cut back on the food in order to add the drink, you'll wind up with mighty slim pickings at mealtime.
- The calories you get from alcohol are like those in sugar—empty. They contain nothing that is good for you. A comedian once suggested that they should produce a vitamin gin so you could build yourself up while you tear yourself down. As a matter of fact, it has been seriously suggested that healthy additives should be put into alcoholic beverages, but the government won't allow it, probably on the theory that it would only encourage people to drink more—hardly a national goal.
- Drinking is not recommended on the HCF diet because it seems to cause a rise in triglycerides. Dr. Anderson is realistic enough to know that his patients sometimes drink. He figures that if the drinking isn't excessive and the patient is neither overweight nor high in triglycerides, then drinking doesn't completely destroy the virtues of the HCF diet.
- For someone following Bernstein's high-protein, high-fat plan, alcohol presents a particular problem because it can keep proteins from being converted to glucose. Since this diet uses protein rather than carbohydrates as the main source of glucose, an alcoholic drink at mealtime can be dangerous.
- Alcohol is risky for diabetics taking either insulin or oral hypoglycemics because it can interact adversely with them. Here's another of those ubiquitous "check with your doctor" situations.

- For diabetics who are overweight, the problem is that alcohol tends to lower inhibitions, and your formerly well-controlled hand may start straying toward the cocktail snacks and popping them into your mouth. Therefore, you get calories upon calories—those of the alcohol plus those in the snacks.

- For insulin takers, the danger with alcohol is compounded first— and this is true for all diabetics, according to Dr. Leo P. Krall—if you eat while drinking, alcohol will push your blood sugar up; but if you *don't* eat while drinking, alcohol can lower your blood sugar. So you can get in trouble in both directions.

- To keep blood sugar normal, the body can manufacture sugar from its stored animal starch (glycogen), a process that is called gluconeogenesis. Alcohol blocks gluconeogenesis. Insulin also blocks release of glucose from the liver. So an insulin-dependent diabetic who has not eaten for a while—thus depleting the body's glycogen supply—and who then drinks alcohol is in danger of experiencing a blood-sugar plummet to the insulin reaction level. If, in addition, alcohol makes you forget to eat at the time you need to, you could begin to slur your speech and stagger your gait and perhaps even pass out. The average policeman—in fact, the average anybody—would be likely to consider you a common drunk, as they like to call them, and treat you accordingly. The treatment of a common drunk is not the kind of treatment that brings about a raising of the blood sugar.

- Alcohol also reduces the body's ability to fight infection, and since diabetics are already more susceptible to infection it's unwise to further reduce the defenses.

- Oh, yes, and there's always the liver damage that accompanies long-term excessive drinking. But then, we aren't here discussing long-term excessive drinking for diabetics. *Nobody* condones that.

If, after all this diabetes temperance society haranguing, you've decided you do want to have a drink now and then, to fit alcohol into an Exchange List diet, you count it as a fat. For example an ounce and a half of hard liquor is two Fat Exchanges. A four-ounce glass of dry wine is also two Fat Exchanges. Beer is one Starch/Bread Exchange plus two Fat Exchanges, because it contains carbohydrates as well as alcohol.

When you come right down to it, you're probably getting the answer here that you get from a doctor who will take an occasional drink. Done intelligently in moderation, it's not ghastly for you and your diabetes. We both drink (intelligently and in moderation) and consider a glass of wine something that embellishes a meal and we're happy to say that it's much less of a forbidden fruit than it has been in ages past. In fact, studies have found that moderate consumption of alcohol may reduce the risk of heart attacks, strokes, and other diseases. Research has indicated that red wine provides more health benefits than does white wine, beer, or liquor. This was first brought to the attention of the American public back in 1991 when *60 Minutes* broadcast their segment "The French Paradox." The paradox was that although the French consume fattier foods, they have a much lower per capita rate of heart disease than Americans. The likely cause of this was the red wine that the French regularly consume with their lunch and dinner. According to a *Wall Street Journal* report of a study in *Nature,* red-wine grapes contain fruit pigments that inhibit the production of a peptide that stimulates hardening of the arteries, thereby reducing the risk of coronary heart disease.

Derek Paice, a research engineer and type 2 diabetic for over seven years, achieved excellent control with diet alone by scientifically testing the effect of different foods on his blood sugar. In *Diabetes and Diet: A Type 2 Patient's Successful Efforts at Control,* a thirty-six-page booklet with more than forty graphic charts showing his experiments, he explains the method that allowed him to obtain control without pills or insulin. Why are we talking about this in a section on alcohol? Well, one of the discoveries of Paice's dietary experiment is the beneficent effect of red wine, more specifically merlot, on both his blood sugar and his cholesterol. He now incorporates a 4-ounce glass with dinner. Although this is what happened to just one man, it has some good food—and drink!—for thought for any type 2. His booklet can be ordered from: Paice & Associates, Inc., 36181 East

Lake Rd. #147, Palm Harbor, FL 34685. It is $10 including shipping and handling.

But that's not the whole of the wine story. *The Wine Spectator* of November 15, 2001, described a real cork-puller of a Danish study reported in *Archives of Internal Medicine*. The study focused on Danish adults—363 men and 330 women aged from twenty-nine to thirty-four. Ninety-four were wine drinkers, 90 were beer drinkers, 340 were wine and beer drinkers and 169 were abstainers. The study found that wine drinkers had a slightly higher average IQ than the other categories and also that the wine drinkers were less neurotic, less anxious, less depressed, less delusional, and even had fewer psychotic thoughts than their beer-drinking counterparts." The wine drinkers were found to consume "fewer servings of alcohol per week than the other drinkers—and were less likely to abuse alcohol." The study even went so far as to say that "wine drinkers tend to be smarter, wealthier, and more stable psychologically than beer drinkers and nondrinkers." Of course, the conclusion wasn't that the consumption of wine instilled all of the above positive traits in people, but rather that these traits are "associated with better health, and that may explain the connection between drinking wine and having a lower risk of certain diseases." Even so, as you sip your glass of red wine, it does give you a warm glow to think what an outstanding human being you must be.

Still, if you decide for any reason that you'd rather not drink alcohol, you could try a mineral water with a twist of lemon or a dash of bitters at cocktail time. Or if you want to have a drink with very little alcohol but with lots of oral gratification, you could try a spritzer made with a small amount of wine and a large amount of club soda or mineral water.

Choosing one of the above options can have several advantages. You are, after all, drinking *something,* so you don't feel odd or different or left out when others are swilling away. (We've often found that with many of the restrictions of the diabetic diet, giving up certain things is not the hardest part. The hardest part is feeling you're not doing what everyone else is doing and it makes you feel like an oddball. It's a pity we all have these tuggings toward conformity, but we do seem to.) Then, too, a designer mineral water such as Perrier or Pellegrino is usually as expensive as an alcoholic drink so you won't feel you're incurring the wrath of the waiter or bartender by taking up the space of a paying customer without buying anything. Mineral water is also now very much the drink of those beautiful people who want to stay slim and alert and who shun anything alcoholic, sugary, or chemical-laden. And, finally, there's the simple fact that drinking pure water is excellent for your general health and if we can incorporate water drinking into a social ritual, it's all to the good.

A Story with a Happy Ending

Broadway musical comedy star Elaine Stritch had a drinking problem. Big time. She also had a diabetes problem and it kept getting bigger-time because of the drinking problem. Finally it came to pass that, as a *New York Times* article about her put it, she had a "near fatal diabetic attack." (Acutely severe hypoglycemia or low blood pressure.) At any rate, the "attack" and a note of advice and encouragement from Noel Coward ultimately caused her to totally quit drinking. Her career has flourished since then, culminating in her 2001 one-woman show, *Elaine Stritch at Liberty.* Among many rave reviews for her performance was that of *New York Times* theater critic Ben Brantley, who wrote: "She is tall and blonde, with skyscraper legs and klieg-light eyes, and she has the approximate energy quotient of a supernova in midexplosion. And—oh, did I mention?—she is 76."

Could that diabetes wake-up call have helped bring her to this triumph? Probably not, and yet again . . .

THE WATER CURE; A NATION OF GUNGA DINS

It seems that half the American population is worried that they're not drinking enough water. You see them toting their water bottles everywhere like Kipling's legendary water-bearer. You see them swigging away in their cars, on the street, at movies, anywhere at all. And you see them lined up nervously and impatiently at restroom doors. Why this national obsession with drinking water?

It beats us. While we agree that most of us should drink more water than we do, are our bodies really "starving" for it and do we really need the requisite minimum of eight eight-ounce glasses a day? Some water gurus even go so far as to say it should be eight to *ten* eight-ounce glasses. And isn't it a little suspect that everybody from a near-anorexic fashion model to a 350-pound pro tackle gets the same prescription? A variable consumption suggestion is to drink half a gallon for every 100 pounds of body weight.

But not to quibble, just what are excessive quantities of this everyday elixir supposed to deliver unto you? Browsing through the Internet, that great source of health information, some accurate, some questionable, and some ridiculous, you find that drinking more water will: give you mental clarity; make you feel better; give you more energy; help you lose weight (assuming that you're overweight); make your body less susceptible to bacteri, viruses, and pollutants; prevent constipation, irritable bowel syndrome (which increases your risk of hemorrhoids and colon cancer); and diminish headaches, grogginess and dry, itchy skin. One of our favorites is the warning that heartburn, arthritis, back pain, angina, migraines, colitis, high blood pressure, diabetes (?!), depression, loss of libido, chronic fatigue syndrome, lupus, multiple sclerosis, and muscular dystrophy are indications that your body is desperate for more water.

If you explain that you drink a lot of other liquids during the day: tea, coffee, soft drinks, and a little wine with dinner, don't these help the dread dehydration problem? Not so! The analogy is given that if you've been directed to wash your wall with water what will happen if you decide to use coffee or Pepsi Cola or cabernet sauvignon instead. Besides, they tell us, caffeine and alcohol are dehydrating agents that will suck away your body's already limited store of water.

The fact that you never feel thirsty doesn't cut it with the water-bucket brigade because having a dry mouth is not the first but the last signal that you're getting dehydrated. If you wait for that to happen, you're asking for trouble.

Barbara, who's always willing to try anything that isn't harmful and might be beneficial, tried to go onto the eight-glasses-of-eight-ounces-a-day plan and failed miserably. It was too boring and time-consuming and hard to remember how many glasses she'd had, especially if she forgot to write them on the calendar. Her situation was another of those "If it can't be done it won't be done" roadblocks. In her case it couldn't be done. But truth be told, although she didn't make the eight-glass minimum and didn't really feel any different with the increased water, she is trying to drink more—around four glasses is what it works out to.

So what are you to do? You don't want to jeopardize your health but you can't fit all that water into your life—and out of your body? You may be relieved to find that a recent *Los Angeles Times* article calls into question the magic number of eight eight-ounce glasses of water a day. ▸**DiabetiLink #11:** The Water Tide May Be Turning (See p. 275)

But, according to. Peter A. Lodewick, M.D., author of *A Diabetic Doctor Looks at Diabetes,* more than the quantity of water we drink, we should be concerned with its quality. "Although tap water may be safe for many healthy people," he says, "it may be dangerous for those with weakened immune systems . . . certainly people with complicated and uncontrolled diabetes might . . . be susceptible to some infectious agents formed in tap water." For this reason, Dr. Lodewick says bluntly, "The only type of water that seems to be fit for consumption is distilled water, which is water that is virtually free of any minerals, chemicals, or biological contamination." He points out that "distilled water is an excellent solvent" that could "dissolve mineral deposits that have accumulated on artery walls and that often lodge in tissues as one gets older. This could partially reverse the arthritis and joint disease that these mineral deposits cause." His conclusion is that since most diabetes complications are a result of accelerated aging effects of diabetes, drinking distilled water is particularly important for people with diabetes to help "ward off the disease's premature aging effects." His deeds follow his words. He has a water distiller in his home.

THREE FOR OBLIVION: THE ANTINURTURERS

These couldn't in any way be called food since they provide no nourishment. On the contrary, they do not build health; they only tear it down. But since they are put into the body, we'll consider them here. Consider them and dismiss them with contempt.

Smoking: The Unbearable

Okay folks, brace yourselves for a rant. We are unalterably opposed to smoking. In fact, we hate it. Fortunately, we are not alone in our intolerant attitude. While drinking doctors may approve of an occasional cocktail or glass of wine for diabetics, even a chain-smoking doctor (and there are fewer of them every day—you might say they're a dying breed) will not give a diabetic the go-ahead on smoking.

Smoking has been called the number-one preventable cause of death. Whatever verbal pussyfooting the tobacco industry engages in, the fact is you run a hugely greater risk of getting chronic bronchitis, emphysema, and lung cancer if you smoke. Unfortunately, just because the gods have chosen to plague you with diabetes does not mean you have a built-in immunity to other diseases.

As a diabetic, however, you have special reasons not to smoke. Smoking causes a narrowing of the blood vessels and this makes you even more susceptible to those cardiovascular problems that are already lurking about, ready to pounce on a diabetic. Because of this blood-vessel constriction, smoking also further complicates another complication of diabetes—poor circulation. As you know, poor circulation can help bring about such diabetic delights as gangrenous toes.

And are you ready for another negative effect of smoking? There is a greater risk for retinitis, the condition that can lead to blindness. Blood-vessel constriction leads to a lessened blood flow, which in turn causes a decrease in oxygen content of tissues (hypoxia), which ups the chances for developing that blindness-inducing retinitis.

We've also noticed that smokers always seem to be nervous and twitchy. Does the nicotine make them so or are they just nervous and twitchy waiting for their next nicotine fix? We don't know, but these nervous twitchers are obviously under stress. (They also put others around them under the stress of having to watch them.) And stress is exactly what we're trying to deliver diabetics from.

If you gather from the above that we're against smoking for diabetics, you gather correctly. In fact, if you're a smoker and you ever visit either of us, please check your cigarettes at the door.

If you don't smoke, don't start. It's not sophisticated; it's stupid. It is, as former HEW secretary Joseph Califano called it, "slow-motion suicide." It's also said by some to be a harder habit to break than heroin. If you already have the vile habit, do whatever you have to do to break it, even to the point of paying for a service, such as Smokenders or Schick, to help you. (In some areas, the American Cancer Society has free stop-smoking programs.)

End of rant.

Marijuana

Our first objection to marijuana is the same as our objection to smoking. After all, you do smoke it—unless, of course, you make it into Alice B. Toklas brownies, in which case our objection is the same as our objection to sugar. In addition to that, marijuana has the inhibition-reducing and judgment-suspending qualities of alcohol, the problems of which we've already discussed. It also shares with alcohol a tendency to weaken the body's immune system. In addition to *that,* with marijuana usually comes the munchies, prompting you, almost uncontrollably, to eat everything in sight, and there goes the diet.

In addition to *that,* marijuana may cause high blood sugar by breaking down and releasing the body's stored glycogen. In addition to *that,* it's illegal. And, finally, in addition to *that,* it's still an unknown commodity as far as what it does to your long-range health. Those who maintain that it's less detrimental than alcohol may well be wrong. It may merely be that alcohol has been used so extensively and its effects have been studied for such a long period of time that we're more aware of the damage it does. It may be years before the ill effects of long-term marijuana use are discovered, and then it may be too late.

When you do all of this addition, it's clear that marijuana should be subtracted from any diabetic's list of drugs.

But despite all these negatives, we are positively in favor of marijuana for medicinal purposes for relief for people with cancer and AIDS and other painful diseases.

Cocaine

At first we weren't even going to bring up the subject of cocaine. After all, what person in his or her right mind who already has one expensive habit—diabetes—would want to take up another? (We once heard cocaine defined as nature's way of telling you that you have too much money.) But, according to statistics, there are *many* people not in their right minds. An estimated five million Americans are regular cocaine users and thirty million have tried it at least once. Therefore, we'll present you with some of the potential hazards of cocaine use.

Cocaine has been proven to cause nasal-passage damage, including loss of the sense of smell, as well as constriction of blood vessels, quick rise in blood pressure, angina, irregular heartbeat, a rupturing of the aorta, heart attacks, strokes (both the paralyzing and killing variety), atherosclerotic heart disease, drowning from a sudden accumulation of fluid in the lungs, liver damage, seizures, tremors, delirium, psychosis, impotence, and, in pregnancy, fetal damage or death, and infant abnormalities such as low birth weight, and a panoply of neuro-behavioral disorders. Is that enough for you? If not, try death, which can occur during your first experimentation with the drug.

Diet: The Art of the Matter

A SHIFT TO THE RIGHT HALF OF THE BRAIN

During the 1960s, scientists studying the structure and working of the brain developed the theory that different sides of the brain have different talents and perform different tasks. The left side is the logical, rational, analytic, objective, and intellectual side. So far we've been mainly using the left side as we learn the basics of diabetes control—the *science* of diabetes. Now we're concentrating on the right side, the intuitive, free, imaginative, creative, mystical, holistic side, and that's the side with which you practice the *art* of diabetes. Of course, diabetes requires the use of your whole brain all the time. You can't have good control and good health without the left half and you can't have good times and a good life without the right. But at any given time, one side or the other dominates, depending on the circumstances. Now's the time to let your right half take center as we investigate the pleasures of the table and how to get them.

THE JOY OF COOKING

You may feel that you can't fit "scratch" cooking into a schedule already crammed with diabetes activities. But stay. Cooking not only provides the additive-free, nutritious food you need to maintain optimum health and diabetes control; it also can be a mental-health booster and stress reducer in itself.

The writer John Irving says, "If you are careful, if you use good ingredients and you don't take any shortcuts, then you can usually cook something very good. Sometimes it is the only worthwhile product you can salvage from a day. With writing, I find, you can have all the right ingredients, give plenty of time and care, and still get nothing. Also true of love. Cooking, therefore, keeps a person who tries hard sane."

Also true of diabetes. How often have you tried hard and still come up with a 250 blood sugar? Cooking keeps you sane, but only if you don't go about it insanely. If you attack your cooking in a frenzy, trying to get it over with as quickly as possible, you'll build up stresses that even the most perfect diet will have trouble counteracting. Working quietly and concentrating on what you're doing makes cooking creative, enjoyable, and sanity promoting.

THE FARMER IN THE PARKING LOT

One very good cook of our acquaintance says that the secret of cooking is to get the best, freshest ingredients you can and do as little to them as possible. Of course, growing your own ingredients makes for maximum freshness, but if you have no place for a garden and no terrace for containers, there's something that can be your dietary salvation: farmers' markets. In the last decade they've been springing up all over the place in our part of the country, and they may be springing up in yours if you look around for them. (We were once in New York City and ran across the one in Union Square.)

At these markets you'll find a stunning array of the best and brightest of local seasonal produce plus such things as one-day-old eggs and home-cured olives, and, of course, plants and flowers. The price will almost always be less than, and the fruit and vegetables always twice or three times as fresh as, in the supermarket.

Shopping in one of these open-air markets is also a joyful experience and a great stress reducer. The people (both buyers and sellers) are friendly and eager to tell you how to cook things you may not be familiar with and to offer new suggestions for the use of old vegetable friends. One Frenchwoman told us five new ways to prepare leeks while we were lined up to buy them.

If you don't know if there are any markets in your area, try calling the local newspaper. That's where we've discovered most of those we go to. It's worth doing a lot of seeking to find something so life- and spirit-enhancing.

HEARTS AND FLOWERS

The dining atmosphere can be almost as important to your control as the diet. Mealtime should be a soothing respite from the stresses of the day.

Practicing what the Hindus call "one-pointedness"—concentrating on the enjoyment of the meal—is vital. A radio or TV shouting out the day's mayhem report is not conducive to mealtime tranquility. Neither are family arguments. A calm atmosphere helps you savor your food, and when you really taste what you're eating you can achieve a feeling of satisfaction with less food and thus will be less tempted to break your diet with a second helping.

Another way to leave the table not feeling hungry and yet not overeating is by eating more slowly. Although we don't advocate "Fletcherizing" your food—chewing each mouthful thirty-two times (once for each tooth), as was advocated by turn-of-the-century food faddist Harold Fletcher—we do feel it's a good idea to retreat from the frenzied chomp-and-gulp style of so many people in our hurry-up society. Aside from not really getting the maximum pleasure out of your meal, when you eat too fast your body doesn't have a chance to send your brain the "I am full" signal and you tend to eat more than you should or leave the table feeling hungry.

Snail Power

Once we were fortunate enough to spend the summer in France. When we came back and dined with family and friends, we found that we were still calmly eating when the rest of the group was finished and drumming their fingers on the table with impatience. What had happened was that we were in the European dining mode, eating about half as fast as we normally did in this country.

Now there is an actual international "slow-food movement," founded in Paris in 1986 by journalist and gourmet Carlo Petrini, and developed in Italy as a response to the arrival of Italy's first fast-food restaurant, a McDonald's in the historic Spanish Steps area of Rome. The movement, symbolized by a snail, has grown to 65,000 members in forty-five countries. Not only do they advocate slow eating and savoring at the table, but they also foster the production of local products and taking the time to prepare them with care. Italians being Italians, they have taken the movement even further by establishing a network of "slow cities," which has grown to thirty towns. The entrance of each slow city displays the movement's logo: a snail crawling past an ancient and a modern building. Not only do they support organic culture and local cuisine, but they protect green spaces, build bicycle and pedestrian paths, limit car traffic, and don't allow neon lighting or car alarms. They even encourage businesses and schools to adjust their hours to allow for a long midday meal with friends and family. You can become an official member of the movement by contacting the US Slow Food Movement on the web at info@slowfoodusa.org, or write to 434 Broadway, 7th floor, New York, NY 10013 USA, phone: 1-212-965-5640 or fax: 1-212-226-0672. Or you could just display a picture of a snail or a snail ceramic in your home and declare your own "Slow House." You'll quickly (!) discover what a difference it makes in your dining and your whole outlook.

Another thing to remember in your Slow House is that candles and freshly cut flowers and other table enhancements contain no calories. Nor does it raise your blood sugar to arrange the food attractively on the plate. On the contrary, these very aspects of beauty at mealtime, along with a calm and loving atmosphere, tend to turn off the day's adrenaline and make control easier.

SOLO BITE

Joke: A man died and went to heaven. God greeted him and asked if there was anything he wanted. "As a matter of fact, yes," admitted the man. "I haven't eaten in a while and I *am* a little hungry."

"Fine, I'll go get dinner," said God.

While the man waited he passed the time by looking down below at the devil's domain, where the hellions were at their evening meal: caviar, beef Wellington, pheasant under glass, pâté de foie gras with truffles, the most luscious fresh fruits and vegetables, beautiful homemade rolls, fresh-churned butter, wine flowing like water—everything anyone could want. The man was really salivating by the time God returned.

And what did God give him? A dry cheese sandwich and a glass of water.

"Gee, God," said the disappointed man, "I hate to complain, but how come they're eating all those terrific things down there and all you give me is a cheese sandwich?"

God sighed. "It didn't seem worthwhile cooking for just the two of us."

It's no joke that people living alone often feel it's not worthwhile cooking for just the one of them. Or if they do cook, it's as one friend of ours reported: "I knew I'd hit the gastronomic skids when I found myself standing by the stove eating dinner out of the frying pan."

Since 20 percent of America's households are now composed of one person and since many of these are older people who are into the years of high diabetes incidence, it stands to reason that there are a lot of people who are going to be tempted not to bother cooking "all that food" on the diabetic diet. This can cause real problems with their diabetes, especially since people in the maturity-onset (type 2) category can often control their diabetes with diet alone if they follow the diet carefully.

June, who over the years of diabetes has often been a solo biter, always carefully presents herself with well-balanced meals based on the diet. For her, this was a big general-health change for the better from her pre-diabetes days. Then she seldom planned meals in advance and would just drift vaguely toward the refrigerator and eat whatever she happened to find there. Not only does she prepare the diabetic diet now, but she treats herself the same way she'd treat a guest, presenting the meal as attractively as possible, pouring herself a glass of wine, listening to pleasant music, trying to make the meal a soothing, restoring experience in every way.

The American Diabetes Association publishes *Quick and Easy Recipes for One.* (You can double the amounts in case God drops in for dinner.) This has one hundred recipes that are, indeed, quick and easy and diabetically appropriate to boot. You could, of course, cook recipes for four or six and freeze the leftovers for later meals.

In a sense, diabetics living alone have an advantage in following the diabetic diet in that they can eat exactly what they should eat without feeling they're "imposing the diet" on hapless family members. Admittedly, though, it is more pleasant to dine with a companion (if he or she is a *pleasant* companion) than it is to dine alone. Loneliness can bring on depression, which can in turn cause you either to lose your appetite or to eat too much (or to eat things that are bad for you, like sweets) by way of compensation. And none of that is good for your diabetes.

If you live alone, why not get together with other solo biters and start a dining club to meet for dinner once or twice a week, taking turns fixing the meal or each bringing a dish? If you belong to a diabetes group, maybe you could find a diabetic dining buddy and enjoy the challenge of fixing right-on-the-diet meals together.

THE FAX OF RESTAURANT LIFE

It's always a great comfort to be able to plan your restaurant meal ahead of time, and now it's not just possible, but easy. All you need is access to a fax machine—at work, home or a neighbor's.

You simply call the restaurant where you're planning to go and ask them to fax you a copy of their menu. This they gladly—and usually promptly—do. In fact, the request is so common now that they don't bat an eye or flap an ear at the request. The first time we did this we thought we were clever devils to have come up with such a brilliant and original idea. But the restaurant responded to our request so readily and matter-of-factly that we realized a lot of others had thought of it before.

It's terrific to be able to sit at home quietly and calmly mapping out your perfect meal. Then when you arrive at the restaurant you can decisively place your order.

And speaking of decisiveness, June has found another advantage to having a menu faxed to her. Often when we go out to a restaurant with friends, the menus arrive and everyone is laughing and scratching and chatting and having something to drink. As a result, they pay little or no attention to the menu. The waiter arrives asking if the table is ready to order. Everyone says some variation on the "No" theme. The waiter leaves. Now people deign to look at the menu but no one can make up his or her mind. Again the waiter arrives. Again he's sent away. Finally everyone decides what they want, but the waiter is nowhere to be seen. He's pretty much given up on this table. After a certain amount of attention-getting hand-waving and signaling (epitaph for a waiter: "God finally caught his eye") he returns to finally take the order.

During all this prolonged ballet of ordering, June has been sitting there scrunching her vitals because she's taken her insulin. (Humalog = 15 minutes to action time) and doesn't want to stuff down bread and spoil her real dinner.

With the faxed menu, before the party leaves for the restaurant, June can suggest what fun it will be to select our dishes before leaving, then we can relax and enjoy each other's company without having to fret over what we're going to order.

It works and that's a *fax* fact.

New trend: The last two times we requested menus by fax they asked if we had access to the Internet. We did and they gave us their website address. There we found an attractive display with an extensive write-up of the restaurant, its location and hours, and menus for all the meals they served. We expect this will catch on.

UNFAIR FARE SHARE

The Chinese have their centuries-old way of dining. Large platters or bowls with portions for four to six people are placed on the table with serving utensils and each diner receives a small plate. Once we had a Chinese meal in Japan, and there was a large lazy Susan in the center of the table. You could spin it around to serve yourself from the different dishes. The great thing about this dining system is that you can sample many dishes, choosing more or less of one or the other according to your personal taste—or diet. The Chinese still eat in this unique family style as you well know if you go to Chinese restaurants in this country.

Now, centuries later, Americans dining out have put a strange new spin on the Chinese way of eating, usually to the detriment of diabetic diners. Here's how it works: type 1's who must eye-measure their food to balance it with their insulin dosages and type 2's who need to control portion size and fat and calories select from the menu the food that precisely fits their dietary needs. Then, voilà, when the appetizer arrives, the new American sharing habit kicks in. Everybody wants to taste your dish and have you taste theirs. The *New York Times* of November 10, 1999, points out that plate-passing is now immensely popular, almost *de rigueur,* as fast-forked friends dip into your food and you're supposed to dip into theirs. Sometimes your plate returns to you with almost nothing left (you chose better than they did!). A slight variation on this theme is when your neighbor diner insists on giving you a bite of their serving with, "Here I want you to try this. It's super-delicious." Then, out of politeness, you're forced to offer him or her a piece of your cherished entrée.

All this creates a dilemma if you know and like and want and *need* what you ordered and if their stuff is detrimental to your diabetes control—too much carbohydrate, fat, sugar, etc. Letitia Baldrige, the etiquette guruess, says sharing food is a pet peeve of hers. "It's a regression of manners back to the caveman days. . . . It's exceedingly unappetizing, not to mention sloppy and slovenly and ungracious." We'll drink to that, plus our own: "It's unfair, unhealthy (what germs those forks might bear!), and even antidiabetic.

We favor un-sharing, but how to do it without seeming un-friendly and selfish? June finally despaired of her problem of dining with some old and beloved friends who were addicted to plate-passing and its associate system of ordering a single appetizer (their selection) and then having all four in the party share it.

Her solution to these dining dilemmas was a little daring the first time she tried it, but it went over very smoothly. She announced dur-ing the menu-reading period that she saw what would be exactly right for her, but was worried because she would have to consume her entire portion herself due to her dietary restrictions. No one bat-ted an eye or battered the reluctant sharer. The other three, as was their habit, stuck their forks in each other's food and June ended up a happy chomper, her palate satisfied and her blood sugar in control.

Another strategy she uses applies to dessert. Often the table orders one dessert for everyone to share. ("Go ahead, June, try it, a little bite won't hurt.") She announces that she *really* prefers an espresso. This is no lie, she's a coffee devotee and self-appointed connoisseur. This seems to make them happy as they work their way through their pecan pie or tarte tatin or tiramisu.

We'll end this share war by quoting our favorite French chef, Julia Child. This ever-outspoken one, counsels, "Announce at the begin-ning of the meal, 'This time, let's not share.'" Her other technique, only possible if you're Julia, herself, is to decree that everyone at the table order the same thing—the only sure way of keeping other people's forks where they belong.

RESTAURANT ROULETTE

The greatest challenge to eating healthy meals comes as you cross the threshold of a new restaurant and are presented with an unfamiliar menu. You have to read it as carefully as if you were trying to decipher a code (you are!), interrogate the waiter with the dedication of a member of the medieval Inquisition court, and as you place your order, turn the phrase "on the side" into a verbal tic that pops out as frequently as "you know" in some people's speech patterns.

The dangers you're trying to avoid in restaurants are too much sugar, too much fat—and just plain too much. Restaurants are as bad as commercial food processors when it comes to throwing in gratuitous sugar to "make food taste better." Indeed, sometimes they pose a double threat because they use commercially processed food that contains sugar to begin with and then they compound the felony with their own wanton sugar spoon.

Although sugar can find its insidious way into anything, including vegetables and mashed potatoes, salad dressings and sauces are particularly risky. Even when you've grilled the waiter and he swears there's no sugar in something, you may not be safe. He may not know that a healthy (?!) amount of sugar has been thrown in. We recommend *always* getting salad dressings and sauces on the side whenever possible, and if you're unsure about whether or not they're laced with sugar, we offer another suggestion from the ever-ingenious Dr. Dick Bernstein of the low-carbohydrate–diet fame: carry Tes-Tape or Diastix with you and discreetly dunk them into suspect substances. If they register below ½ percent glucose they're probably okay.

Here we want to insert a special word of caution about ordering soft drinks in restaurants. If your diet Coke, or whatever, does not arrive in a can or bottle, beware. One survey showed that about one-third of the time the diet drink was the real thing. Only Tes-Tape or Diastix will tell.

When it comes to fat, it's truly amazing how much a restaurant can serve up. Naturally, as a diabetic you'd never order deep-fried (or shallow-fried) anything, but restaurants like to throw fat on everything and often throw it on in a way that's difficult, if not impossible, to remove. Toast and English muffins come soaked in butter. Hot rolls frequently arrive with pats of butter melting over their brows. Vegetables swim in butter or, in the fancier restaurants, drown in hollandaise sauce. Meat suffocates beneath gravy; fish is buried in sauce. Never assume that *any* dish is going to arrive in a pure, unfatted state. On the side. On the side. On the side.

Incidentally, besides too much sugar and too much fat, restaurants generally give you (or, rather, charge you for) too much food, period. Both diabetics and nondiabetics who care about their weight and health need to have Great Dane–sized doggie bags to carry out all the leftover food. Our solution is, whenever possible, to eat out at lunch rather than dinner. Or, if you're on a trip when you must eat all your meals out, try to eat the main meal at lunch and have the lighter meal (such as soup or salad and a sandwich) for dinner. This has several advantages. At lunchtime, restaurants serve less food and charge less for it; the price of lunch in the best restaurants in town may be only around half what you'd pay for larger amounts of identical food at dinner. You can, therefore, enjoy haute cuisine and elegant ambience without breaking either your diet or your bank account. On top of that, if you eat your main meal at lunch you have a much better chance of walking or working off any excess sugar, fat, or calories you may have been unable to avoid.

FAST-FOOD CHAIN DINING

Once, when we were musing on the idea that you can be taking excellent care of your diabetes but neglecting your health, the example occurred to us that you could follow the standard Exchange List diabetes diet while eating all your meals in fast-food chains. In that case, you would indeed be taking care of your disease but neglecting your health, because fast-food chains are very big on all those things you should avoid—sugar, white-flour products, salt, fat (most of it saturated or hydrogenated), and miscellaneous chemicals. They are also very small on those things you need for a healthy diet—fresh fruits and vegetables, fiber, whole grains.

Off and on the chains make attempts to healthy-up certain of their foods The sad truth is that they often wind up dropping the healthier selections because people don't order them, preferring the old familiar, less healthy ones.

Helen Oswalt, editor of the *Keeping in Touch Newsletter for Scripps Whittier Diabetes Education/Support Diabetes Groups* recently ran a list of what horse-racing circles call "The Best of a Poor Field." These are the things you should select if you find yourself hungry and on the premises of a fast-food dispensary.

- **Burger King:** B-K Broiler sandwich (without mayonnaise) = 390 calories, 8 grams of fat. You might add a small side salad or a few slices of tomato if they are available.
- **KFC:** Tender Roast Sandwich (without sauce) = 270 calories, 5 grams of fat; Corn on the Cob (without butter) = 150 calories, 1.5 grams of fat.
- **McDonald's:** Chicken McGrill (without mayonnaise) = 340 calories, 7 grams of fat; regular hamburger = 270 calories, 9 grams of fat.; Chicken Caesar McSalad Shaker with fat-free vinaigrette = 130 calories, 2.5 grams of fat.
- **Subway:** Ham, Turkey Breast, or Roast Beef 6-inch sandwich = less than 300 calories, 4.5 grams of fat (less fat than that if you have it without cheese, mayonnaise, or oil); or Veggie Delight = 200 calories, 2 grams of fat.
- **Taco Bell:** Bean Burrito = 370 calories, 12 grams of fat; grilled chicken or steak soft taco = 200 calories, 7 grams of fat (each).
- **Wendy's:** Grilled Chicken Sandwich (without honey mustard) = 310 calories, 8 grams of fat; baked potato = 310 calories, 0 grams fat (sour cream and chives for the potato = 70 calories, 7 grams of fat).

As you can see, this is a very limited selection and not a complete nutritional analysis (For example, there is no listing for carbohydrates and fiber.) But if you have access to the Internet, you can enter www.kenkuhl.com/fastfood. There you can click on Fast Facts and find a list of over 1,300 menu items from twenty-four restaurants with their nutritional analysis.

Another good source for fast-food information is *Nutrition in the Fast Lane,* a pocket-sized booklet providing full nutritional information on 2,400 menu items from forty-nine fast-food and casual dining places. You can order this for $8.45 (including shipping) from Franklin Publishing, Inc., 310 N. Alabama St., Suite 350, Indianapolis, IN 46204; phone: 1-800-634-1993; e-mail: franklinpub@fastfood facts.com.

THE DOUBLE-CROSSING OF THE SALAD BAR

Salad bars can be hazardous to your health. People breathe heavily over them, scattering droplets laden with bacteria and viruses. They fondle the vegetables with their grubby hands, and leafy ingredients are often sprayed with allergy-activating sulfides. But worst of all, although you think you're having a virtuous diet meal, you can get loaded with calories from the dressing, or dressings, as the case may be. One study showed that the average person takes in more calories from a salad-bar lunch than they'd get in a standard meat and potatoes meal! Solution? Avoid, if possible, this barbaric practice.

THE MIXED BLESSING OF THE SUNDAY BRUNCH

The Sunday Brunch is fast becoming an American institution, but we can't give it an unqualified hallelujah. The most popular and widespread form of it is the buffet or, as June calls it, the groaning board—with an emphasis on the groaning. While it is a good thing to be able to wander about selecting the foods that are right on your diet, the temptation is always there to select more than you should, especially in the dessert sector. But even if your willpower remains strong, it becomes rather boring for you to eat your allotted portions and have to sit there twiddling your thumbs while others gorge and gorge and go back to gorge some more.

Barbara has a different reason for not being totally enthusiastic about Sunday Brunches. There's the champagne that is usually served and even if you just drink one glass, that, combined with all the carbohydrates that abound, makes you logy dopey for the rest of the day (carbohydrates make you sleepy—even without champagne). A much better way to spend Sunday is to have a light lunch after sleeping late or attending church, whichever is your habit, then going out for a walk or a bike ride or a tennis game; something vigorous and energizing that will give you pleasure as well as a workout.

Barbara's been lobbying for a different Sunday meal. It could be a called lupper, a combination of lunch and supper served in the late afternoon or early evening. Your muscles will feel pleasantly relaxed from your day of fresh air and exercise and if champagne and carbohydrates made you a little sleepy then, that would be no problem. You could retire early, say after seeing *60 Minutes,* and arise the next morning full of vigor and ready for the challenges of the week ahead. So far, no restaurant has taken Barbara up on this idea, but perhaps if you joined with her we could start a grass-roots movement.

Exercise

When Barbara took a course in acupressure at Los Angeles Valley College a while back, it actually turned out to be a course in general health as well. (It was based on the book *Touch for Health Program* by chiropractor John F. Thie.) One of the main goals of the instructor was to get everyone in the class, whatever his or her age or physical condition, into an exercise program. By way of motivation she told a little story. It seems there was a guru who always gave the same advice when people came to consult him about their problems.

"I am sad," one would say.

"You ought to exercise more," was his response.

"I have no energy," another would say.

"You ought to exercise more."

"I can't sleep nights."

"You ought to exercise more."

We could play guru like this with all your diabetes-associated problems.

"I am overweight."

"You ought to exercise more."

"I am underweight."

"You ought to exercise more."

"I am always hungry."

"You ought to exercise more."

"My blood sugar is always high.

"You ought to exercise more."

"I keep having insulin reactions."

"You ought to exercise more."

"I am depressed and discouraged over my diabetes.

"You ought to exercise more."

"I want to get off the pills."

"You ought to exercise more."

"I have poor circulation."

"You ought to exercise more."

We could go on and on. No matter what ails you physically or emotionally, exercise helps. Strangely enough, it even helps contradictory conditions. Type 2 diabetics often have difficulty losing weight and juveniles sometimes can't gain. Exercise can help both problems.

SOLVING WEIGHTY PROBLEMS

It's not illogical that if you exercise more you will burn more calories and lose weight. But many overweight type 2's argue that exercise just increases their appetites and that at best they stay the same weight and at worst they gain. Wrong. Studies done by nutritionist Jean Mayer have shown that vigorous exercise actually *suppresses* the appetite. When we were researching our book on biking (*Biking for Grownups*), we found that people on long bike tours had to be reminded that they should eat carbohydrates at regular intervals even if they didn't feel hungry. And they usually didn't feel hungry because of the body's failure to give the eating signal during sustained exercise.

Dr. Mayer made another interesting discovery. People who lose weight through exercise tend to be better at keeping it off than those who take if off through dieting. We read an explanation for this in *Fit or Fat* by physical-fitness expert Covert Bailey, who says a well-exercised body that doesn't have too much fat on it handles calories

differently; it burns them at a high rate no matter what you're doing—even sitting still or sleeping!

We won't *guarantee* you'll lose weight with exercise. Something
else—equally good—may happen. You'll lose fat, which will be replaced with muscle. Since muscle weighs more than fat, your weight
may remain the same but your measurements and appearance will
improve vastly.

Your diabetes control is also likely to improve, because, as we
mentioned earlier, overweight type 2's often have *too much* insulin in
their blood (hyperinsulinemia). The excess insulin is floating around
along with excess sugar because obesity has made these persons' cells
insulin-resistant, and the insulin can't unlock the cells and let the
glucose in. The pancreas keeps getting high blood-sugar signals and
produces more and more insulin in a vain attempt to bring the blood
sugar down. With exercise and a reduction of fat in the body, the
cells become more receptive to insulin so that the sugar can get into
the cells more easily and the pancreas can stop overproducing insulin. Therefore, you have the paradox of better control with less insulin. This is one of the reasons why overweight diabetics who reduce
the fat stores in their bodies through exercise and proper diet can often get along without insulin or pills and, in fact, get rid of almost all
their diabetes symptoms.

EXERCISING CONTROL

Exercise has special benefits for lean, insulin-dependent diabetics, too.
Those of you who have a regular program of sports activity have
probably noticed that when you exercise you can put on needed
weight, and when you don't you tend to lose it. Why does exercise
have the opposite effect than it has on overweight non–insulin–
dependent diabetics? The answer is that with exercise the leans stay in
better control and their food is totally utilized by the body instead of
being thrown out and wasted as sugar in the urine. Also, when glucose
from the diet cannot be adequately utilized, the body starts eating itself up, a kind of do-it-yourself cannibalism. Here's the experience of

a diabetic physical-education professor we know: "I'm a rather lean, muscular 180 to 185 pounds. If I don't exercise I lose weight. My control is affected and my sugar levels increase. I then must return to my high activity level to gain it back."

Another benefit is that physically active, insulin-dependent diabetics find they not only have less high blood sugar but less low blood sugar as well. In other words, exercise has a stabilizing effect on blood-sugar levels. The explanation of this is simple: (1) exercise helps glucose get into the cells (we like to think of it as a kind of "invisible insulin"), and thus helps reduce high blood sugar, and (2) it also helps the body build up its store of animal starch (glycogen) in the muscles and liver; this glycogen can be converted to glucose whenever needed, so active insulin takers have a good internal reserve of glucose for hypoglycemic emergencies and, hence, are less subject to low blood sugar.

EXER-HIGHS

Exercise simply makes you feel better all over—body and mind. This may be because for a while you're escaping from the pressure cooker of life as you exercise. And then again it may be the release of a hormone called norepinephrine. This hormone makes your spirits rise. A British medical team headed by Dr. Malcolm Carruthers found that only ten minutes of vigorous exercise was enough to double the body's level of this happy hormone and put a person in a better frame of mind.

Besides a rise in spirits, you get another kind of high from exercise. Dr. Ethan Sims and his wife, Dorothea, in their "Dialogue About Diabetes and Exercise" in the *ADA Forecast* for July/August 1974 quoted one of their friends describing his running experience.

I also experience a type of high which has not often been commented on. The initial exhaustion of a run wears off in around five to ten minutes. About a half hour later, a gentle warmth begins to suffuse the lower limbs, which complements a state of complete physical relaxation. The sensorium is sharpened and thinking becomes more acute. A total sense of well-being, which may last three to four hours, permeates the event.

This high from exercise is for real. Diana Guthrie pointed out in her diabetes-education classes that exercise activates the body's endorphin system, and do you know what endorphin means? The morphine within. So you're getting yourself a perfectly delicious natural high with no harmful side effects. Well, maybe one. Just like the real stuff, the body's own morphine is addictive. Active sportspeople will tell you that when they have a day without their exercise fix they suffer withdrawal symptoms and become nervous and irritable.

But don't worry. Your addiction is what psychiatrist Dr. William Glasser calls a positive addiction, one that is good for you, one that makes you a stronger, healthier person in mind and body—and a better-controlled diabetic.

A MOVING MEDITATION

Another way that exercise makes you feel better is that, like meditation, it cleans your mind of the distressing mental debris—or it should if you're concentrating on your sport the way you ought to. If you're playing tennis, for example, and start thinking about the errands you're planning to do later or a fight you had with your spouse rather than about your game, you might as well walk off the court, because you're bound to lose. On the other hand, if your mind is totally on the tennis, you'll get a double benefit: your mind will be cleaned out and you'll have a much better chance of winning.

The same is true of all sports. Downhill skiing is a particularly good example. Since it's such a basically unnatural sport—you have to lean out away from the hill when every fiber of your being wants to lean into it and cling—you have to really concentrate on what you're doing or *splat!* You also need to be on the alert for hazards (human—especially snowboarders—and otherwise) on the slopes. But another factor that makes skiing so great for ridding your mind of your troubles was summed up by a British businessman we once met in Lech, Austria. He said that skiing is the only sport he really likes. "When I'm up there on the slope," he said, "I forget about all of my business worries. I'm so bloody frightened that all I can think of is how I'm going to get down the hill in one piece." Skiing will even make you forget you have diabetes. Guaranteed.

FRIENDS INDEED

Exercise is also a great way to meet people. If you take up a sport, you soon acquire a new set of friends who share your enthusiasm. What's best about this for a diabetic is that your sports friends are the right kind of friends, the kind who will reinforce the healthy lifestyle you want to follow. They will be the kind who don't want to carouse around all night because they've got an early morning golf reservation or they're taking off at dawn to go hiking. If you meet someone in an aerobics class and decide to go to lunch together, it's not likely he or she will want to gulp down french fries and pecan pie with whipped cream. They've worked too hard to get in shape and won't want to blow it in a few moments of dietary indulgence.

Warning: There are some exercise fanatics who have what one psychologist termed "yuppie bulimia." These are people who spend half their time doing extremely strenuous exercise so they can spend the other half stuffing down food. Obviously, these are not the kind of friends you would seek out, since they would be a bad influence on your diabetes in two ways.

YOU GOTTA HAVE HEART

At one American Diabetes Association meeting where we were carrying on about the virtues of exercise for diabetics, a gentleman in the audience asked if he really needed to exercise since his job involved physical labor. Probably yes. There are very few jobs that give you the right kind of exercise for optimum diabetes health. The only one we can think of offhand is that of the mail carrier who walks at top speed (a mile every fifteen minutes), rushing through the swift completion of those appointed rounds. And how many of them do that?

While all manner of exercise is better than doing nothing, the kind of exercise that produces the above-mentioned marvelous benefits for diabetics is aerobic exercise. Aerobic exercises are those that condition the heart, lungs, and blood vessels and lower cholesterol and triglyceride levels while increasing the body's ability to utilize oxygen. In other words, aerobic exercises ward off such cardiovascular problems as heart attack and stroke that plague the modern world in general and the diabetic population in particular.

Aerobic exercises are done:

1. *Continuously.* This means that the exercise must be done without stopping. If you're going to exercise for half an hour, you don't stop once during that entire half hour.

2. *Rhythmically.* A rhythmical exercise is one in which the muscles are contracting and relaxing on a rhythmical basis. Walking, jogging, running, hiking, cross-country skiing, swimming, bicycle riding, jumping rope, roller skating, rowing a boat—all these activities are rhythmical. You are moving yourself from one place to another under your own power in a steady manner. You can see that games like golf and tennis do not qualify—there is too much stop and go, which breaks up the rhythm.

3. *In intervals.* This word describes how you exercise continuously for your fifteen minutes, half hour, forty-five minutes, or whatever. You work fast and then you alternate with an interval at a slower pace. Swim fast for two pool lengths, then slow for one; fast for two, slow for one—slow enough not to have to stop completely.

4. *Progressively.* This means that your exercise becomes progressively a little more difficult. When your body adjusts to one level of workload, you increase the amount you do. The trick is to progress in a lot of little steps.

5. *For endurance.* This word simply says that you're doing an endurance type of program, one that lasts more than five or ten minutes. Endurance activities improve your cardiovascular fitness, and that's the most important kind of fitness for a diabetic.

ACCESSIBLE AEROBICS

The following aerobics are readily accessible in that you can do them right out your front door—or even in the privacy of your home.

Running and Walking

As the Buddha said, "The only constant is change." Nothing has been more constant than our changing attitude toward running. When we wrote *The Diabetic's Sports and Exercise Book,* we said, "Jogging and running bore the very sweatsuits off us." Then when it came to the original edition of this book, we had become jogging/running enthusiasts—not fanatics the way a lot of runners are, but sweetly reasonable enthusiasts doing a mile to a mile and a half almost every morning. This had come about partially as a result of what we learned when June was trying to cure her chronic headaches. Dr. Otto Appenzeller in New Mexico discovered that running is an effective headache therapy. He also found that running creates the relaxation response not too unlike that attained by yoga, hypnosis, meditation, and the like—a toning down of the autonomic nervous system. And, as every dedicated runner will tell you, your whole life changes along with your body when you embark upon a rigorous running program. One study showed that runners are more likely to make major dietary changes for the better than participants in any other sport. Running also gives you a lot of exercise in a short period of time. It's true that you burn as many calories walking a mile as running a mile, but it generally takes longer. And time was of the essence for us, as it is for everyone these days. Running was also in style. Everyone was reading Jim Fixx's running book and everywhere you looked people were stretching against trees and telephone poles and jogging and running and panting and sweating and training for marathons. As advocates of exercise, we could hardly not be runners.

Then styles changed. Jim Fixx's fatal heart attack while running dampened the enthusiasm a good bit. Actually, since he had a family history of heart trouble, his running probably gave him several extra years of life. Still, it provided a good excuse for people who wanted to stop running anyway. The medical reports also started coming in about the damage to knees and ankles from the incessant pounding, especially when the running was done on a hard surface, as it generally was, and for runners who were over forty, as many were. Some type A personalities (the intense, hard-driving, competitive sorts whom Dr. Meyer Friedman described in his book *Type A Behavior and Your Health*) found that they were out running with a stopwatch, pushing for a faster time, a greater distance, putting greater pressure on themselves, just as they do on the job. Running, instead of reducing stress, was creating more.

We gradually climbed onto the new bandwagon of walking not running. Unless you have a passionate love for running, we suggest that you follow in our footsteps. Walking is the one sport that virtually anyone can do without risk. In fact, as one doctor put it, "It's impossible to walk too much." And the Joslin Clinic unequivocally states in its manual, "Walking is the best exercise for your feet." We all know how important foot care is for people with diabetes. And if you'd like a professional athlete's endorsement of walking, take Hall of Fame tennis champion (and diabetic!) the late Bill Talbert. On days when he didn't play tennis, he made it a point to walk forty to fifty blocks. He died at the age of eighty.

Here's the definitive endorsement of walking and other nongrueling physical activities. A study of 17,000 Harvard alumni revealed that you don't need to do arduous sports like running marathons to reap the lifesaving benefits of exercise. Men who pursued such moderate activities as walking, climbing stairs, and sports that used 2,000 or more calories a week had death rates one-quarter to one-third lower than their more sedentary fellow graduates. The lifesaving benefits of exercise peaked at expending 3,500 calories a week. Burning more calories in exercise than that number in some cases proved to have a slight detrimental effect.

To determine how many calories you're burning in a particular activity so that you can reach the magic 2,000-a-week number, see ▶**DiabetiLink #11:** Chart of Calorie Expenditures p. 277. One conclusion of the Harvard study was that a daily brisk, three-mile walk will keep you fit and healthy and increase your life expectation.

You may even want to try racewalking. It really moves you along, and all the wiggling motion is a great reducer and toner. It's also enough of a recognized sport to be in the Olympics. One night, a friend took Barbara out to a racewalking class. When they got there, there was a big crowd in the stands and a lot of people milling about. "Gee," mused Barbara, "I didn't know there was that much interest in racewalking. This sport is really catching on." It turned out that indeed there *wasn't* that much interest in racewalking. This was an all-comers track meet and racewalking was only a small part of it. About fifteen people were standing together in the racewalker corner. Two or three were experienced competitors; the rest, like Barbara and her friend, were there to learn and—unbeknownst to them at the time—compete.

After about ten minutes of instruction, they were told that they would be walking a race. (That really chilled their marrow, but there was no way out.) Everybody lined up and then were off on a walk of four times around the track. In no time at all the experienced people lapped the learners and then lapped them again. After what seemed an interminable time, the only "competitors" left were Barbara and her friend. As the athletes were jogging and pacing around the periphery of the track getting ready for the 100-yard dash, a voice boomed over the loudspeaker, "The 100-yard dash is delayed. There are still two walkers on the track." That chagrin speeded them up a little, but it still seemed forever until they crossed the finish line. But as luck would have it, despite their dismal showing, Barbara and her friend took a second and third in their age category.

Racewalking is easy to learn. After this brief and harrowing indoctrination, Barbara was able to teach June, and whenever not too many people are watching, we break into the racewalk wiggle and it's truly a workout. If you're interested in trying it, look for a class—preferably one that doesn't involve a public competition at the end. Racewalkers are an extremely dedicated and evangelistic lot and they're delighted to sign on converts. If you can't find any classes or evangelists in your community—and even if you can—you should read *The Complete Guide to Racewalking Technique and Training* by Dave McGovern, an excellent book for the beginner that you may be and the elite competitor you may become. Another good book is *Racewalking for Fun and Fitness* by John M. Gray. It's now out-of-print but available used on Amazon and half.com and in libraries. Gray tells you exactly how to do it and inspires you to action. Incidentally, although he is also a medal-winning runner, he considers walking the better sport.

But whether you decide to go for running, jogging, racewalking, or just plain vigorous walking, as Dr. Joan Ullyot of the Institute for Health Research in San Francisco says, "The hardest step . . . is the first one out the door." If you're ready for this first step, this is how we suggest you go from there.

First, we suggest investing in a good pair of running or walking shoes. Fortunately, there are stores selling all kinds of these all over the country. Unfortunately, not all salespeople are knowledgeable about how to help you select the right kind of shoes and/or how to fit them correctly. Shop around and ask a lot of questions. One warning: please, we beg you, don't use tennis shoes for running or walking. They don't position your feet properly and are designed more for lateral than forward motion. Also, they don't protect you from the jars and jolts of the road, sidewalk, track, or ground. With the wrong shoes, these jars are transmitted throughout your body, creating trauma and stress.

Aside from the shoes, you can wear anything that's loose, comfortable, and appropriate to the weather.

Speaking of weather, don't let the weather provide you with an excuse. If you let the heat or the cold or the rain or the snow or the wind or the hail or the smog or the earthquake stop you, you'll wind up never running or walking at all.

When should you run or walk? We prefer mornings. Excuses seem to be easier to come by in the evenings, and if you exercise in the morning you can enjoy its benefits the whole day.

The "safe" time for insulin takers to exercise is after meals, when the blood sugar is on the rise; it reaches its height one to one and a half hours after a meal.

Before you go out you should always warm up with a few stretching exercises for the leg muscles—see the section of this chapter called "A Stretch in Time." As part of your warm-up routine it's also a good idea for the first few minutes of your outing to walk if you're a runner and to walk slowly if you're a walker. You should do the same thing for the last few minutes to cool down. And never take a hot bath or shower immediately after you exercise. You should wait for the blood to return to your innards from your feet and legs before you draw it away to the surface of your skin with hot water.

When you first begin your program, do it for only fifteen minutes. We prefer to work with time rather than distance. If you have a goal of a certain number of miles, you may try to run or walk faster to get them over with and get back to some project that's hanging over your head. This destroys the whole conditioning and relaxing aspects of the routine.

A good basic rule is to walk as fast as possible and run as slowly as possible. A slow run is at a "conversational pace." This means you're running slowly enough to carry on a conversation without getting out of breath.

And that's all there is to it. Keep at it every day (or with one or two days a week off), gradually increasing the total time and the amount of that time you spend running or walking. Your body will tell you when to make the increases: you may work up to half an hour or even an hour, and then again you may not. Don't stress yourself over it. Just do what feels right.

You may wonder what to do with your mind while you're doing all this with your body. Well, what you shouldn't do is stew over your problems and sort through all the things you should be doing instead of "wasting your time" exercising. That builds up the kind of stress that negates the benefits of the exercise. One thing you can do is combine meditation with your run or walk. Chant your mantra, count your exhalations, or do whatever best cleanses your mind of its incessant woe-churnings (see chapter 10 on meditation). Or just look around and enjoy nature or people watching. You'll see a lot of things you miss when whizzing by in a car.

The Great Indoors

Although it's lovely to be out in the fresh air doing your exercise, sometimes the air isn't fresh. In Los Angeles we often have a smog alert and you're sternly advised not to go out to exercise in it. Or the air may be too fresh and freezing cold. Or in northern parts of the country in the winter there may not be enough daylight available to do your exercise if you're trying to fit it in before or after work. Or, especially if you're a woman exercising alone, you may feel a bit uneasy out walking or running by yourself in this hazardous world. Or it may be that you haven't quite worked your body into the kind of shape that you want to display on the city streets or country roads or athletic fields or tracks. In all of these cases, the answer may be indoor exercise. Here are a few possibilities.

Jumping Rope

This takes up very little space and takes almost no equipment (you can just use an old piece of clothesline). But if you want to get fancy, there are jump ropes available that rotate within the handles. You can get your heart rate up quickly with a vigorous period of rope jumping.

Aerobics

There are a lot of VCR tapes available for aerobics. They do a good job of keeping you motivated and moving and charting your heart rate so you don't overdo or underdo. There are also good TV aerobic programs. If you have a VCR, you can record them to use whenever it's convenient for you. In both of these cases, look for the "low-impact" kind that doesn't do harm to your joints.

Rebounding

Doing aerobics on one of those rebounders or minitrampolines is an exhilarating exercise and, since the rebounder gives with each step, you can do the standard non–low-impact aerobics without joint problems. This is Barbara's favorite great indoors aerobic activity. The *Hooked on Aerobics* program from the Brigham Young University that appeared on PBS is her favorite. The routines are entertaining, varied, and sound; and the people doing them are attractive but not extreme-bordering-on-weird in their appearance and spandex swathed the way some aerobic performers are. It is also available on audiotape. Both are available on the Internet from http://creativeworks. byu.edu or by calling 1-800-962-8061.

Exercycles

These range from the basic to the many bells and whistles versions. (Note: every bell and every whistle raises the price, sometimes to stratospheric heights.) Many people like the Airdyne because you get more bang for your energy-expenditure buck since you exercise both arms and legs (and even a little upper torso). The recumbent bikes are gaining in popularity in our multitasking society because you sit up on a comfortable chair and can read or even write. Many of the fancier models give you heart-rate monitoring and can be preprogrammed for such speed and effort variations as intervals, summit, hills, plateau, triathlete (!), and random.

Cross-Country Skiing Machines

These *really* give you a workout. It has been said that the cross-country skier is the world's most physically fit athlete. This includes both muscular and cardiovascular fitness. These machines, however, do not come without some disadvantages: they're on the expensive side and take up quite a bit of space, both during use and in storage.

Elliptical Cross Trainers

These are currently the newest, trendiest item on the exercise equipment scene. They are sometimes described as a cross between a cross-country skiing machine and a stairclimber. Their advantages are that they give you a total body workout in a short time without the stress and jarring impact that can cause injuries. They're also easy-to-use and burn a whole bunch of calories. Even people with arthritis of the hips, knees, and ankles, who ordinarily can't run, can use these. The bad news is that, at this point, the elliptical cross trainers for home use are very expensive and, according to *Consumer Reports,* they don't hold up under repeated use. Better to use one in a gym or health club until the home models improve—or until they go out of style in favor of a newer, trendier kind of equipment.

Treadmills

When you talk about being on a treadmill, you're referring to a not-too-pleasant, grueling life, but when it comes to exercise equipment, treadmills are the most popular kind—at least so say the treadmill manufacturers. They do have many advantages: they allow you to walk or run when the outdoor weather doesn't permit it, they give you a good cardiovascular workout at your own speed and fitness level, they're easier to master than many other exercise machines—after all, most of us have been walking since the age of two—you can do a lot of things while exercising on them (study language tapes, watch television, etc.) Treadmills range from the simple to the complex. The latter giving you steepness level adjustments, electronic feedback displays of speed, time, and distance, many have preset programs for you to follow, and heart-rate monitors, And here goes the old refrain again: the problem is that the good ones are expensive and the cheap ones are not good. P.S. They take up a lot of space.

Rowing Machines

These are good for working out the upper as well as the lower body. They can often be tucked behind a sofa or under a bed so they don't intrude on your interior decor. There are even videotapes available that give you a rowing routine complete with peripheral outdoor scenery.

Penny Foolish

In purchasing your exercise equipment, buy the best you can afford or maybe even a little better than you think you can afford. Ignore those super-bargain ads in the paper for brands of equipment you've never heard of. These are the kinds that are so unsatisfactory to use that they wind up hidden in a closet or gathering dust in the garage. Even if you stick to using them for a while, they often break down before you do. Especially beware of cheap exercycles and dinky little rebounders with feeble springs. Thrift note: Many people with the best of intentions purchase very expensive pieces of exercise equipment and soon find they hardly use them—if at all. After hanging their clothes on them for a while, they decide they're just cluttering up the room and sell them via newspaper ads or at garage sales. You can pick up some good bargains that way. If you shop and inspect the piece of equipment carefully, a well-known used brand in good condition is better than a new piece of junk.

Women's Choice

In selecting a sport (indoor or outdoor), women should remember that unless part of your exercise is load-bearing, it doesn't help prevent osteoporosis, something we all want to avoid. Therefore, if your sport of choice is swimming, biking, exercycling, or rowing, remember to throw in some of the others that will get you on your feet and carry you around. Variety is more fun anyway.

GOALS AND GUIDELINES

Gary Scherer, when he was executive director of the Center for Heart and Health Improvement and director of Cardiac Rehabilitation at the Daniel Freeman Hospital in Inglewood, California, devised a very sensible exercise program for total health for everyone. With a few modifications, it fits beautifully into a diabetic's exercise regime. He believes you should practice your exercise three times a week, or every other day. (We feel many young diabetics can and should exercise regularly every day.) The way the program goes is:

1. Fifteen minutes of stretching and flexibility exercises.
2. Five minutes of cardiovascular warm-up; moderate to brisk walking is ideal.
3. Thirty minutes of cardiovascular exercise—jogging, running, swimming, bicycling, jumping rope, aerobics, or folk dancing, to name a few.
4. Five minutes of cardiovascular cool-down—reduced activity to allow the body to recover properly.
5. Enough sport and game activities to satisfy the competitive and social spirit.

The general guidelines for following your exercise program include:

1. Exercise regularly. The benefits of exercise cannot be stored; sporadic exercisers are subject to increased risks of injury.
2. Train, don't strain. Always exercise within your capacity. It is usually better to exercise longer than for brief periods at high intensity.
3. Time is in your favor. Take at least one month to get in shape for every year out of shape.
4. Exhale on effort. Breathe out during the effort cycle of muscular exercise (that portion of muscular exercise during the strenuous phase).
5. Avoid isometric exercises (those that pit one muscle or part of the body against another or against an immovable object). These can significantly raise the blood pressure and place additional strain on the heart.
6. Don't exercise during illness. This may aggravate the problem, particularly with infectious diseases.
7. Never end with a sprint. The demands of a sprint after cardiovascular exercise may exceed the safe capacity of the heart.

8. Don't withhold drinking liquids. Adequate water replacement during exercise is necessary to compensate for water loss through sweat and respiration.

9. Don't exercise through pain. If pain persists, call your personal physician.

10. Avoid extremes in temperature. Exercising in environments of extreme temperature or quick temperature changes after exercise, such as a very hot or cold shower or sauna, is dangerous.

11. Use sweat clothes properly. Sweat clothes are for warm-up, cool-down, and cold weather. Improper use can cause marked increases in body temperature, leading to heart palpitations or even death. Rubberized suits to promote heavy water loss are completely inadvisable.

12. Proper shoes. Weight-bearing exercises can place strain and trauma on the joints and muscles. Well-fitting and cushioned footwear can minimize or eliminate this. Proper choice of exercise surface can be beneficial.

13. No alcohol prior to exercise. Alcohol and many drugs constrict the vessels of the heart, and the increased demands for blood and oxygen during exercise cannot be met.

14. Reduce exercise level at high altitude. The amount of oxygen available to your lungs and bloodstream is reduced and thus your exercise level must be reduced.

15. Avoid marked fatigue. It's not normal to be fatigued two hours after an exercise period.

16. Increase motivation. Participate in different physical activities; exercise with a group of friends; change locations.

17. Sweating is normal. Sweat is a normal by-product of metabolism of moderate to heavy exercise and helps cool the body.

18. Stop cigarette smoking. The harmful effects of smoking reduce heart and lung capacity.

Besides these general guidelines, we have a few special ones for diabetics.

Additional Guidelines for Diabetics over Forty

Get a stress test. This will tell you how much exercise you can safely do. Barbara decided that since she's always telling others to get a stress test and since she's past the year of demarcation, she ought to take her own prescription. After getting wired up and trudging the treadmill, she was told by the doctor that "anything you *can* do won't hurt you." That is to say, if she *could* run the Boston Marathon or ski in the Vasaloppet cross-country race or swim the English Channel she wouldn't get a heart attack if she did it.

Even if you don't intend to get into an active exercise program—although we can't imagine you wouldn't after the heavy hype we've given you—you should still get a stress test. Dr. George Sheehan, the famous proselytizer of running, says that a person who sits around doing nothing all the time is the one who needs a stress test the most because inactivity is one of the greatest stresses on the body.

Just to add the spice of medical controversy to the stress-test advice, the *New England Journal of Medicine* for August 2, 1979, reported a study that concluded that "the ability of stress testing to predict coronary-artery disease is limited in a heterogeneous population in that the prevalence of disease can be estimated through classification of the pain and sex of the patient." The news media immediately translated this as "those expensive tests are worthless."

One of June's former doctors, an internist who specialized in cardiology and diabetes, translated it more moderately this way: "Essentially they are saying that the degree of accuracy [of the stress test] is directly proportional to the type of patient population that is being tested. They are also emphasizing that there is no substitute for an extremely accurate, complete history and physical examination. In summary, submaximal stress testing is useful only as a diagnostic adjunct to complete evaluation by a competent physician."

You might ask your own doctor for a translation.

Alternate your exercises. After forty it takes longer for your muscles to repair themselves after exercise, so it's best not to do the same exercise two days in a row—except, of course, walking, which you can't do too much of. For the more vigorous exercises, though, it's best, for example, to jog one day and ride your bike the next, swim one day and jump rope the next, or however you want to alternate.

If you're over fifty, it may be best to exercise only every other day. Again, though, this doesn't mean you should be inactive. You should keep moving, walking, climbing stairs instead of taking elevators, and being a generally vigorous person every day.

Do something. No excuses. Even if you're in your eighties or nineties, even if you have a heart problem, there are exercises you can do to improve the circulation in your feet and legs. These exercises act as an insurance policy against the dire things that can happen to diabetic toes, feet, and legs in advanced years. Figure 2 shows a series of exercises known as Buerger-Allen exercises. They should be performed before you get out of bed in the morning.

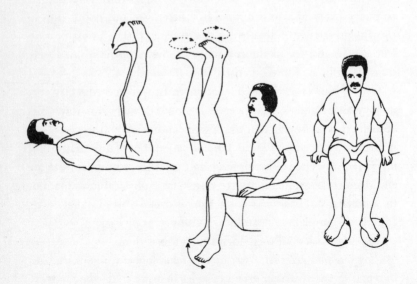

FIGURE 2. *Buerger-Allen Exercises*

Exercise #1

Lying flat on your back, lift your legs until they are perpendicular to your hips. From this position, with the soles of your feet facing the ceiling, move your feet up and down, bending them at the ankle, so that your toes are first pointing to the ceiling and then to the bed. Repeat ten to twelve times.

Exercise #2

While in the same position, make clockwise circles with your feet ten to twelve times. Then make counterclockwise circles ten to twelve times.

Exercise #3

Sit up and hang your legs over the edge of the bed, but don't touch the floor with your feet. Flex your ankles and point your toes first up, then down, as you did in exercise 1. Do this ten to twelve times.

Exercise #4

Now, while in the same position, do the clockwise and counterclockwise circles you did in exercise 2. Repeat ten to twelve times as before.

Additional Guidelines for Insulin Takers

When you exercise more than usual you must either take less insulin or eat more food. Diabetics handle this both ways, although there is a slight edge in favor of eating more because (1) a chance to eat more is always welcome to those on a restricted diet, and (2) a lot of doctors don't want their patients to alter their insulin dosage.

Some very active diabetics we've talked to handle their insulin in just the opposite way. That is, since they exercise heavily almost every day, their usual dosage is keyed to a high level of physical activity. On those few days when they're going to be exercising very little, they increase their insulin.

Another variation is switching to regular or Humalog insulin before each meal, using long-range insulin like Lantus (glargine) as your basal dose. As Dorothea Sims once wrote us, "The advantages of multiple doses when exercising are very great. I just climbed

Camel's Hump, a 4,089-foot mountain, over Labor Day. I couldn't have done it except on three shots of semi-Lente [a fast-acting insulin similar to regular]. So much flexibility and freedom from clock-watching and feeling lively all day long!"

Do not inject insulin into the part of your body that's going to be active. Internists Veikko A. Kovisto and Philip Felig reported that insulin absorption is speeded up at the injection site if intense muscular activity is taking place there. This fast absorption could bring on a reaction. A bowler, therefore, should not inject the bowling arm before playing. A tennis player should avoid arms and legs on the day of a tournament. A skier uses the arms and legs all the time and—especially if a beginner—frequently the rear end as well, so the safest shooting spot on the day of a ski session would probably be the abdomen.

Do not exercise when your blood sugar is over 250 and you have ketones. As Sheri Colberg, Ph.D., says in *The Diabetic Athlete: Prescriptions for Exercise and Sports,* "Exercising with high blood sugar and ketones (indicating a relative lack of insulin in your body) can cause blood sugars to go even higher, which increases the risk of diabetic ketoacidosis (DKA), which can be life-threatening and require hospitalization."

Be prepared for lower-than-usual blood sugar for twenty-four to forty-eight hours after strenuous exercise. Exercise doesn't just lower your blood sugar during the exertion. There is a carryover effect in the evening, on into the middle of the night, and even the following day, because exercise makes the body more sensitive to insulin action. Some diabetics report they have their more severe reactions on Monday after a sports-filled weekend. Be prepared.

ONE HEART BEATS IN THREE-QUARTER TIME

One way you can be sure you're getting enough of your aerobic exercise to strengthen your cardiovascular system, but not so much as to harm it, is to time your pulse. To find out the number of beats per minute, place two fingers on the inside of your wrist or three fingers on your neck on the side just below your jawbone. Using a watch with a sweep second hand, you can—depending on your level of patience—either count six seconds and multiply by 10 or count ten seconds and multiply by 6, or count fifteen seconds and multiply by 4. For example, if you count twenty beats in fifteen seconds, your pulse rate is 80. Practice taking your pulse when you're not exercising until you can do it quickly and efficiently. You have to be fast and efficient enough to take your pulse when you *are* exercising without letting it drop while you fumble around trying to find it.

Gary Scherer recommends bringing your pulse up to 70 to 80 percent of your heart's capacity and keeping it at that level during your whole period of exercise (fifteen minutes minimum). Your heart's capacity is determined by your age and condition. The way to estimate this is to take the number 220, deduct your age, and that equals your maximum heart rate. If, for example, you're forty years old, that would be 220 − 40 = 180. If you were aiming for 75 percent of your heart's capacity, that would be around 135. Exercising at 70 percent capacity is for those of you who have any history of heart disease at all—and you should not do even that much without a go-ahead from your doctor. If you're very out of shape, you shouldn't go over 75 percent; if you're young and in pretty good condition, aim for 80 percent of capacity. The 85 percent is *only* for an athlete in top shape and in training.

If you haven't done any exercising for a long time, you'll be amazed at how little it takes to get your pulse up to its 70 to 75 percent capacity. It may take only a brisk walking pace or even, in some cases, an average or slow pace. But don't be discouraged. If you keep at it, you'll find you're able to do more and more, faster and faster, with the same pulse rate and, voilà, you have good cardiovascular conditioning, a changed metabolism, better control, and another building block for your strong body.

A STRETCH IN TIME

In the list of guidelines for exercise and in our information on running, there was the advice to do stretching before cardiovascular exercises. An ideal way to do this is with yoga.

A diabetic of any age and in virtually any physical condition can benefit from yoga exercises. They are not jarring to the body and you are never supposed to strain yourself to achieve a position. Gradual, gentle, nonpainful stretching is the order of the day. Many people find it hard to believe that yoga exercises produce the wonderful effects they do, because they never leave you feeling exhausted and sore the way many people think exercises are supposed to.

We like yoga exercises for a dual set of reasons. First, they keep muscles and joints flexible, improve circulation, and free metabolism to work better. Second, they reduce mental as well as physical tension. They do this by making you slow down, because the positions are meant to be held for a certain number of counts rather than done in fast repetitions like some types of body-conditioning exercises. Also, yoga instructors (we should say hatha yoga, as that's the official term for the physical aspect of yoga) usually also teach deep-breathing techniques. Remember, we mentioned earlier in the book that fast, shallow breathing is a sign of body stress.

Now to get started with six special yoga positions especially helpful in preparing for aerobic exercises and for overall relaxation. These exercises will loosen all your muscle knots and keep you in condition for those more strenuous blood-sugar–lowering sports like jogging, swimming, bicycling, rowing, and hiking.

When doing these exercises, try to develop a sense of body awareness. As yoga instructors advise, turn off your ordinary mind, the one that's forever churning like a washing machine, and really get into the stretch. Move slowly, smoothly into the stretch. *Be* the stretch. Experience it mentally as well as physically. As you breathe, feel you are actually breathing into the muscle you are stretching.

To do the exercises, choose a quiet room where you won't be disturbed. If the floor is carpeted, use a beach towel over it; on a hard surface, use a thin mat.

Abdominal Breathing (Figure 3)
Lie down on your back with your arms at your sides. Breathing through your nose, inhale, filling your abdomen with air—your ab-

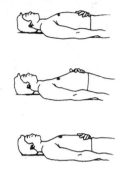

FIGURE 3. *Abdominal Breathing*

domen, not your chest. To be sure, hold your hand on your stomach and make certain it balloons. Practice a few abdominal breaths until you know you're not chest breathing. Now inhale *slowly* through your nose to a count of four. Then exhale *slowly* to a count of six or eight, contracting your abdomen as you do. Repeat this slow, rhythmical breathing ten times.

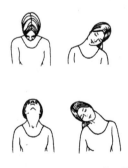

FIGURE 4. *Yoga Head Rolls*

Head Rolls *(Figure 4)*
These are sometimes called neck rolls, because the neck is the part of you that gets the workout.

Keeping your shoulders relaxed, simply drop your head forward with your chin close to your chest and then slowly roll your head in a complete circle, first to the left and then to the right. It's very important to roll slowly. A good technique is to pause several seconds when you get to your shoulder, pause again when your head is hanging backward, and again over your other shoulder. The more snap, crackle, and pop you hear when you do this exercise, the more you need the good it's doing you. When June first did head rolls, she heard a kind of pizzicato string-snapping quartet each time she rolled. Now that she's a regular yoga-exercise disciple, she hears only an occasional bit of crackling.

After you loosen up, you should be able to do at least five head rolls. If they are too much for you at first, just drop your head forward and then drop it backward to stretch the throat. Hold several seconds in each position. Even this simple maneuver is very relaxing.

Chest Expansion (Figure 5)

Stand quietly for a minute with your arms hanging loosely at your sides. Bring them up to shoulder height, stretched out at your sides, bend them, and touch your fingertips under your chin.

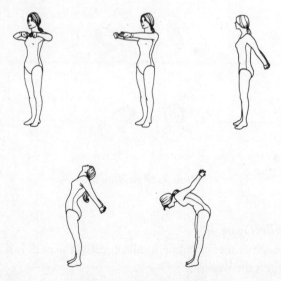

FIGURE 5. *Chest Expansion*

Next, push your arms straight out in front of you and stretch your elbows. Now move your arms—still at shoulder level—around in back of you until you have to stop. Drop them and clasp your hands behind your back.

Keeping your arms as high behind you as you can, bend backward; drop your head back, too, as in a head roll. Hold for a few seconds.

Next, keeping your hands clasped behind you, bring your arms up over your head and bend at the waist until you've brought your arms as far forward as you can. Your head should now be hanging down near your knees. Your neck should be hanging loose. Hang that way for a count of about twenty (make sure your knees are not bent).

Now straighten up slowly and you're ready for the second part of this exercise. Keep your hands locked together behind you. Put your left foot forward. Bend over until your forehead is as close to your left knee as possible without straining. To do this you have to bend your right knee. Feel those left-leg muscles stretch. Hold for a count of about ten.

Now straighten up and repeat with the right leg forward.

Do the entire routine—both parts of it—once more. There you are, revitalized and untensed.

Alternate Leg Pulls (Figure 6)

Lower yourself to the floor and sit with your legs stretched out in front of you. Bend your right leg and, with your hands, bring your heel up close against the inside of your left, stretched-out leg.

Now raise both arms above your head, bend forward, and clasp your left leg as close to your ankle as you can without straining. Pull yourself down as far as you can. That may not be very far at all, but with time and practice you'll get your head far enough down to rest on your knee. Be sure your neck is limp as you hold the position. After a slow count of thirty, let go and straighten up.

Do the same with your left leg bent and your right extended.

Repeat the entire sequence twice.

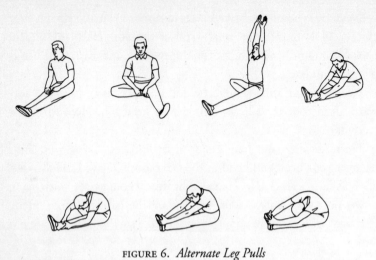

FIGURE 6. *Alternate Leg Pulls*

The Cobra (Figure 7)

Lie flat on the floor face down with your forehead supporting your head and your arms at your sides. Go completely limp. Feel the tightness flow out of every muscle as you lie there playing dead.

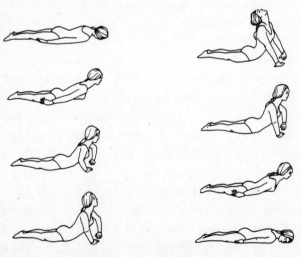

FIGURE 7. *Cobra*

Slowly raise your head and tilt it backward. Lift your upper body as far off the floor as you can without using your hands to help. When you're back as far as you can go without strain, bring your hands in under your shoulders, fingertips facing each other. Slowly push yourself up, your head tilted back toward your toes. Feel your spine arching. Keep your legs relaxed and your eyes closed. When you're back as far as you can go without strain, count to ten.

Lower yourself slowly. Bring your arms back to your sides as soon as you can and let your back muscles be in control as you lower yourself completely to the floor. Rest your cheek on the floor and go limp again.

Do the cobra twice.

The Plough *(Figure 8)*

This is the most difficult of the exercises, but it has a lot going for it. According to yoga teachers, it allows the blood to flow into the thyroid and improves its functioning, and diabetics need all the help they can get with glands. Also, it gets more blood into the brain so that you can think better. However, this exercise is not recommended for those of you with hypertension or an enlarged liver or spleen.

Lie down on your back. Place your hands along your sides, palms down. Slowly lift your legs, knees straight and together (the first

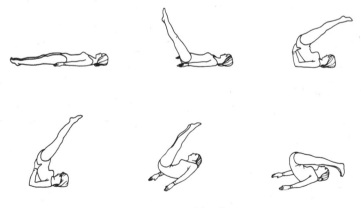

FIGURE 8. *Plough*

few times you do this you may need to bend your knees), and when they're high enough so that it's time to bend at the hips, move your hands up under your hips to brace yourself while you swing your legs into a vertical position. When you're in the correct position, your chin will be almost touching your chest. With your elbows on the floor and your hands bracing your hips, just remain "standing" on your shoulders for at least twenty seconds. (Those who do yoga regularly can hold this position as long as three minutes at a time.)

Now extend this shoulder stand into a plough position. Swing your legs backward with your toes pointing toward the floor. To brace yourself, put your arms on the floor with the palms of your hands down. Keeping your legs straight, lower your toes as far toward the floor as you can without straining or hurting. (Don't worry, you won't break your neck or back, nor will you topple over.) Stay in this position for the count of ten. Feel the stretch all along your spine. Roll out of the position and lower your legs to the floor without raising your head. The more you do this exercise the closer your toes will come to the floor, until they finally touch.

Relaxation Pose (Figure 9)

Lie on your back with your feet slightly apart, falling open naturally, and your arms at your sides with your palms up. Turn your attention to your cheek muscles and gently make sure they are relaxed. Imagine that a hand is gently stroking your hair and relaxing your scalp. Make a point of breathing abdominally through your nose.

Lie in the relaxation pose for at least three minutes. This is a good way to end your exercise session.

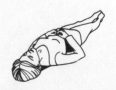

FIGURE 9. *Relaxation Pose*

You may want to sign up for a yoga course at your local community college or recreation department. You can also check the program guide of the educational-television channel in your area to see if it carries either Richard Hittleman's *Yoga for Health* or *Lilias, Yoga and You.*

MUSCLING IN

Just when we thought that with our regular aerobic exercise program we were doing the best we possibly could to promote a strong body, dissenting news started leaking out. The first thing that caught our collective eye was an article in the *New York Times Magazine* (April 26, 1991) entitled "The New Case for Woman Power." No, this wasn't a feminist exhortation for a female takeover of the world. The subject was weight training (also known as resistance training) for women. Not only did it urge women to take up lifting weights because it "accentuates their natural curves, tightens the soft stuff of their thighs, stomach and upper arms and allows them to fit into smaller clothes," but it promised to benefit the cardiovascular system and help increase bone mass, thereby lowering the risk of osteoporosis. Pretty compelling. Enough to start us thinking about going over to investigate a new gym that had just opened about a mile away.

Then, only a month later, there appeared an article in *U.S. News.* This one, called "Muscle Bound," loudly announced that "running, biking and other aerobic exercises are great for your heart, but they're not enough. To stay healthy, you've got to pump iron too." This is because 65 percent of the body's muscles are above the hips and most aerobic exercises do nothing to strengthen and develop them. Only "regular sessions of strength training can prevent and often reverse the progressive withering away of muscles . . . Americans lose at least 30 to 40 percent of their strength and 10 to 12 percent of their muscle mass by the time they are 65."

Strength training does another great thing. When you convert fat to muscle it changes your metabolism so your body burns more calories, a process that helps solve weight problems. And, according to

U.S. News, you can benefit from weight training at any age: "A team of Tufts University researchers . . . put nursing home patients ages 86 to 96 on a weight-training program designed to strengthen their legs. Although most of the men and women suffered from arthritis, heart disease, and high blood pressure . . . after only two months, the participants had doubled, tripled, and quadrupled their leg strength. Two patients developed enough leg strength to discard their canes."

The nondiabetic one among us was sold and ready to race over and join the gym, but the diabetic one still had misgivings. There have been reports over the years that weight training should *never* under any circumstances even be considered by a diabetic. They made it sound as if it would cause all the blood vessels in your eyes and kidneys to pop open and make your toes drop off.

We decided to do research among the more diabetically authoritative publications to see if strength training might actually be possible for diabetics after all and might even have some special benefits for them. We found what we were looking for in the May/June 1990 issue of *Practical Diabetology:* "Weight Training and Diabetes Mellitus," by Richard M. Weil, M.Ed. He certainly had credentials enough to deliver an expert opinion: exercise physiologist in New York City, consultant to the Diabetes Treatment Center at the New York Eye and Ear Infirmary, and consultant to Park Avenue Diabetes Care.

The comment on the article by the editor had particular significance:

A recent article in this publication recommended that people with diabetes not engage in resistance exercise (weight lifting). On publication of that article, I heard strong opinions to the contrary from a number of exercise physiologists. One of them, Richard Weil, was kind enough to put his thoughts into this excellent article, which has been reviewed by your editor, by a retinologist and by a physician well known for his research on diabetes and exercise.

Many young men with diabetes enjoy weight lifting. Over the years, my colleagues and I have preached the party line and attempted to dissuade them from this form of exercise. To the best of my knowledge, we never succeeded in stopping anyone. Mr. Weil's article certainly provides us some reassurance. More important, it provides excellent logical guidelines so that our patients may participate safely in this form of exercise.

The article not only provided some reassurance, but lots of encouragement as well. Weil pointed out that the benefits of weight training for diabetics "include improvements in muscular strength and tone, glucose tolerance, body composition, muscle capillary density, osteoporosis, coordination, self-concept, and strength of tendons, ligaments, and joints." And he agreed with the *U.S. News* article, writing that the metabolism change brought about by weight training aids in weight loss.

He did emphasize that proliferative diabetic retinopathy would be the greatest risk factor in taking up weight training and that weight training should not be started until the retinopathy has been stabilized with laser treatment and the ophthalmologist okays weight training. He also recommended evaluation and close monitoring by an ophthalmologist for those with chronic hypertension and/or moderate retinopathy.

For patients without contraindications, his conclusion was:

Weight training can be a safe and potentially beneficial activity for virtually all patients with diabetes. Physicians should not overlook or dismiss this activity simply because they are unfamiliar with it or do not participate in it themselves. As primary providers of diabetes treatment, physicians should take the opportunity to inform interested patients about the potential benefits of weight lifting and encourage the development and maintenance of strength in patients of all ages.

That was green light enough for us. We marched right over and signed up at the gym and enjoyed (and benefited from) our workouts there, until a combination of crowds in the gym and personal time constraints drove us out. But now we still work out regularly with free weights. And that we fully intend to keep up forever. Our goal is to always be able to lift our bags into the overhead compartments in airplanes during our travels.

One warning we keep hearing about gyms is that you may get worked over by salespeople who want you to sign up for long-term contracts. Don't do it. You may lose interest and stop going (that's what they count on; then there's room to sign up more people) or the gym may be sold to another company that either lets down the standards or refuses to honor the contract you've signed with the previous owners. So beware. Make sure the start-up fee isn't exorbitant, that they have a monthly fee rather than a contract for a year or more, that you can quit at any time with no penalty, and that if you're going to be out of town for a month or more, they'll waive the fee for that period.

If you do join a gym, although there are well-illustrated instructions on each machine, be sure to have (make!) one of the attendants show how to use all the equipment. It makes your workouts a lot easier and safer and builds up your confidence. In our gym, one of the big selling points was that there were always trainers on the floor and you could even have one work with you every time you came in if you wanted to. This selling point turned out to be only that—a selling point. After our initial one hour of instruction, we hardly saw leotard or Avia shoe of the trainer again. We did track her down once to show us a new machine we couldn't figure out for ourselves. Another good rule is to always warm up on a treadmill or exercycle or step machine before you start to work the equipment and then do a cool-down at the end.

Of course, you could always build a complete gym in your home, as did diabetic diabetologist Richard K. Bernstein, M.D. After an extended battle he even managed to get the IRS to approve of his deducting it as a medical expense—which, of course, it was. But don't try this at home unless you have a taste for mortal combat with IRS agents and some good ammunition from a CPA.

When working out, whether in a gym or at home, try not to be too macho about it—and this applies to women as well as men—grunting and groaning and straining to try to lift the heaviest thing you possibly can. For diabetics, this is definitely a rotten idea, and we feel it's not such a hot idea for nondiabetics, either. While on the subject of women acting macho in the gym, we want to assure you that weight training won't make a woman *look* macho. To build up heavy, bulky Schwarzeneggeresque muscles takes the male hormone testosterone. You know, that stuff that makes men want to do such things as start wars and cut in front of people in traffic. Two good books on strength training for women are *The Fitness Factor* by Dr. Lisa Callahan, and *Strong Women Stay Young* by Dr. Miriam Nelson.

Another piece of gym advice for women is to get a friend to sign up with you, especially if you are no longer a teenybopper. It's a little intimidating to launch yourself alone into that sea of youth and beauty and muscle tone. It will also keep you going regularly. Invariably, on the day one of you isn't in the mood to go, the other will be and will drag you along.

So our advice is for you to add weight training two or three days a week to your exercise program. Make it a part of the weave of your life, as a weight-training enthusiast friend put it.

Of course, you should check with your doctor before embarking upon such a program. If he or she says no, ask if there's a specific reason. (For example, "You have proliferative diabetic retinopathy.") If the response is just something like, "Weight training is not a good idea for diabetics," you should refer him or her to the *Practical Diabetology* article. You could even order a copy of that issue of the publication yourself and have it at the ready in case you get a negative response without justification. (*Practical Diabetology,* 150 West 22nd Street, New York, NY 10011. Request Volume 9, Number 3, May/June 1990. It costs $8.00 plus $2.50 shipping and handling.)

Keep in mind that it wasn't too many years ago that diabetics were forbidden by their doctors to take part in *any* exercise. Read tennis champion Bill Talbert's book, *Playing for Life,* and you'll see what it was like back then. Happily, today exercise is universally recognized as a cornerstone of diabetes control.

TWO BRIDGES FROM A STRONG BODY TO A TRANQUIL MIND—AND VICE VERSA: TAI CHI AND PILATES

Tai Chi

Tai chi is a system of exercise for physical health and spiritual growth developed hundreds of years ago in China by Taoist monks. It is still practiced by millions of Chinese people. The 108 basic moves use every part of the body, and the body moves as one unit in a smooth, graceful pattern, almost like floating. Its basic principle is relaxation. Practiced twenty minutes a day, it builds inner strength and has a tranquilizing effect.

In Hong Kong in the early morning you can see people of all ages in parks and plazas overlooking the harbor going through their slow, elegant, daily tai chi exercises with calm concentration. In San Francisco, take a walk from Union Square through Chinatown to Washington Square. There, in front of St. Peter and Paul Church, you'll find the same routine taking place. We're pleased to report that this rewarding practice is starting to catch on throughout the country. This is not surprising, since it develops the physical health, balance, harmony, and mental focusing that we all need in these perilous and stressful times. Now it may be possible for you to find an area in your own town where you can observe it. You might check with the Taoist Tai Chi Society of the United States, 1310 North Monroe Street, Tallahassee, Florida 32303, phone 850-224-5438, e-mail usa@ttcs.org and see if they can give you guidance on where to find tai chi in your area.

There's nothing like seeing the real thing and, if you decide to try it yourself, there's nothing like instruction from a real person, but you can get a good idea of what it's like and learn some of the moves from seeing videos. If you have Internet access you can find these (and reviews of them) by hopping onto your favorite search engine and entering "tai chi." Amazon also has a number of these available. (Of particular value for older people and for those who want to exercise at their desks during the day is *Tai Chi in a Chair* by Cynthia W. Quarta. Another popular favorite despite its put-down title is *The Complete Idiot's Guide to T'ai Chi* by Bill Douglas. If you don't have

Internet access, go to a bookstore or your library and browse the books on tai chi. Books will give you a basic understanding of the practice and probably sources of videos as well.

Pilates

Pilates? What's that? It sounds like a Greek philosopher. No, it's actually an exercise method devised by Joseph H. Pilates (pronounced puh-lah-teez). He was born in Germany, but his family was of Greek origin.

Pilates was in England at the start of World War 1 and, because of his German citizenship, he was interned for the duration. During this time he became a nurse and cared for wounded and immobilized patients. To help them exercise and speed their recovery, he devised exercises with springs attached to their beds. This was the foundation of the exercise equipment—and the program—he later brought to the United States, where he was particularly successful in fitness training and rehabilitating dancers. When he died in 1977, the Pilates torch was passed on to his wife, Clara, and thence to Romana Kryzanowska. Over the years the flame has grown until now it is the hottest exercise concept in town.

We're amazed it took us so long to learn about it, since we always try to look into new trends and often try them out. One of our friends had been doing Pilates for a year and told us of the wonders it had done for her formerly bulging stomach. "That's for me," said Barbara and with this ignoble goal in mind she set off on her Pilates adventure. She loved every minute of it. The exercise hour passed like mere moments, after each session she felt energized, not in the least fatigued. She was never bored—how could she be since in Pilates there are five hundred different exercises, some done on floor mats and others on modern variations of old Joe's spring and cable equipment. And she never once had sore muscles after the sessions. Of course, she was lucky enough to get referred by her friend's instructor to Suzi Lonergan, who was located only three miles from home. Suzi had been trained by Romana Kryzanowska herself, and it shows. If you want to see Suzi in action and get an idea of what a Pilates floor workout is all about, you can or-

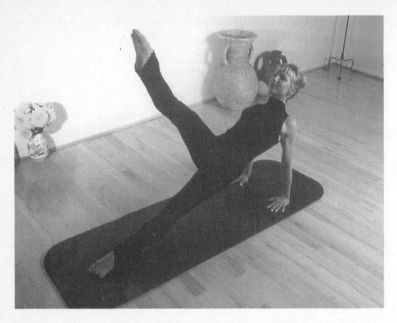

FIGURE 10. *Suzi Lonergan doing Pilates*

der her video from either her website (www.bodypower.la) or her 800 number (866-263-9769 or 866-BODYPOWER). The cost is $24.95 plus shipping and tax (if applicable).

Another way to get acquainted with Pilates is to read two books that Suzi recommends: *The Pilates Method of Body Conditioning* by Sean Gallagher and Romana Kryzanowska, and *The Pilates Body* by Brooke Siler.

Although you can learn a lot from videos and books, you should, if at all possible, have some lessons, preferably at a place where they have the equipment for you to use. Alas, here's another exercise area that's not cheap. According to Joel Braunstein, M.D., writing in the January 2001 issue of *Diabetes Forecast,* "Private sessions may cost anywhere from $50 to $150 per hour." But since, as he points out it's "a method that doesn't demand countless hours of pumping iron or running on a treadmill to achieve an attractive physique . . . a method that pacifies the mind, spirit, and soul," it's worth making an investment in it, and there are semiprivate and group mat classes available at much less cost.

For people with diabetes, Dr. Braunstein cites the reassuring fact that Pilates is an extremely safe activity since the "exercises are mostly performed in a horizontal position on machines or mats, removing the effects of gravity and undue stresses on the spine, back, neck, hips, knees, and ankles."

What benefits are you likely to derive from Pilates? Well, Barbara is a true believer now so you'll need to drain the fanaticism from her benefits list but these are also reported anecdotally by other Pilate-philes: Better posture; weight loss; improved flexibility, coordination, balance, and agility; leaner legs and arms; more toned stomach and buttocks; increased strength; and you may even gain an inch or so in height. To sum up what it does in Joseph Pilates's own words: "In 10 sessions you'll feel the difference, in 20 you'll see the difference, and in 30 you'll have a new body. (Note: This doesn't mean— depending on your gender—Brad Pitt's body or Jennifer Lopez's body, nor does it mean this new body won't have diabetes, but you'll have a new and improved *you* body and that toned up body may be able to handle your diabetes better.)

Another great advantage of Pilates is that you can benefit from it at any age. Romana Kryzanowska is now probably somewhere in her eighties (no one knows for sure). But as Suzi says, "She is ageless! An inspirational force of nature who globe trots, keeping the Pilates flame alight. She works with people in their nineties who were students of Joseph Pilates, and they can still do a full workout!"

But as with anything in exercise, as in life, there are a couple of cautions. Since Pilates is now so trendy, there are many unqualified and inexperienced people wanting to get into the financial action by touting themselves as Pilates instructors. To make sure you're getting a certified and experienced Pilates instructor you should do one of the following:

Call 1-800-4-Pilates and ask for instructors in your area
Check into the website at www.pilates-studio.com

> Call Peak Body Systems (1-800-925-3674) or Balanced Body
>   (1-800-240-3539): both have a list of certified instructors
> Check the two previously-mentioned books (*The Pilates Method*
>   *of Body Conditioning* and *The Pilates Body*) for their list of
>   instructors

For people with diabetes, as with so many physical activities, you should check with your doctor about the advisability of starting a Pilates program. On top of that, Dr. Braunstein says, "If you have retinopathy or neuropathy, review in detail with you health-care team the types of exercises you plan to do. Certain positions that lead to excessive pressures in the eyes are not recommended for those with advanced forms of retinopathy.

We'd like to end with a 1939 quote from Joseph H. Pilates:

This world of ours is in a turmoil and no one is positive of the outcome, and it is now, more than ever before, more practicable and sensible to be in a perfect state of health, both in body and in mind, in order to more successfully confront the problems continually arising.

The whole country, the whole world should do my exercises. They'd be happier. We wouldn't need wars.

So you see, it turns out he *was* a Greek philosopher after all.

PART 2

A TRANQUIL MIND

Now that you've become aware that reducing physical stress through a healthful diet and exercise can also calm your mind, we want to show you how reducing mental and emotional stress will help create a tension-free body.

This intimate connection between mind and body, long recognized by Eastern societies but neglected in the West, is finally coming to the fore in America. Researchers at the Menninger Foundation have proven scientifically that every change in the body produces a change in the mind, and every change in the mind produces a change in the body.

As a diabetic, you may have had considerable experience with the body-mind/mind-body effect. Say, for example, you don't have time to eat your usual quota of breakfast and in midmorning your blood-sugar level drops below 80, into hypoglycemic territory. Now, this is a purely physical happening, but what does it do to your *mental* processes? We don't really have to tell you but, just for review, you get irritable and hostile, confused and indecisive—you "go goofy." Such is the power of the body over the mind. As Kurt Vonnegut has as the continuing theme of his *Breakfast of Champions,* when someone does something outrageous, "his chemicals made him do it."

On the flip side of the body-mind coin, we have for an example a recent event in June's life. It was during the period when she was conducting the high-carbohydrate, high-fiber–diet experiment on herself. Barbara phoned her just before dinnertime and announced, "Guess what? Because of Proposition 13, the college district office has decided we librarians are to keep the library open during Easter vacation week with no extra pay, as voluntary work overload." June hit the ceiling like a rogue champagne cork. That evening, when she took her blood sugar one hour after dinner it was well above 200. At first she couldn't explain this sudden failure of the diet, because she'd been having normal blood sugars for more than a week. Was it too large a potato, the unmeasured popcorn before dinner, extra-sweet strawberries? No. The truth finally struck home. It was her mental rage, the emotion directed against an unfair and arbitrary ruling. And sure enough, after an almost identical dinner the next evening, all was well in blood-sugar land, because all was calm again.

DIABETIC'S CHOICE

How do you go about getting and keeping that calmness even in periods of stress? We're going to consider five different unstressing techniques: biofeedback, progressive relaxation, autogenics (self-hypnosis), meditation, and guided imagery. Only you can choose which ones seem to be right for you; there is no proven difference in their effectiveness. The best results, however, are obtained by combining two or more of these therapies.

A few of the more advanced diabetes-education centers, such as the Diabetes Treatment Center in Wichita, Kansas, early on began offering instruction in the newer methods of reducing physical and mental tension. Diana Guthrie, who worked with her husband, Dr. Richard Guthrie, in the Kansas Center, taught several different stress-reducing techniques in her classes for diabetics and their family members and friends. She advised them to practice any of these methods that appeal to them for five, ten, or fifteen minutes a day for better control of their diabetes.

A final tip is that you get results from these therapies only if you adopt a let-it-happen attitude. Paradoxically, the less you try, the more you progress. How do you manage to soft-sell these therapies to yourself? The directions we've read include such admonitions as "have a creatively expectant attitude" and "plant the seed and let it grow." But perhaps the most graphic and understandable description we've come across is the one that compares the method of performing these techniques to urination: "Just relax and let go."

CHAPTER 7

Biofeedback

. . . .

Of the unstressing techniques, biofeedback is the most palatable to the skeptical scientists. They can't deny the mind-body connection when they see it proved on a machine. The way biofeedback works in a laboratory or hospital setting is that you are hooked up to electronic instruments that feed back information about what is happening inside your body (your temperature, your pulse, your muscle tension, the speed of your brain waves). Using this information, you can learn to control these internal body processes. But you don't have to be hooked up electronically to derive benefit from biofeedback.

Diana Guthrie not only explained the principles of biofeedback to her students but gave them a practice exercise with a thermometer to show them how they can raise the temperature of their hands through the power of the mind. (Warm hands usually mean you are relaxed; cold hands mean you are tense.) You can make your own biofeedback device by purchasing an inexpensive ($3 to $5) mood ring. These were popular in the late seventies and can still be found in novelty shops and on the Internet (look under "mood ring" on your search engine).

The mood ring turns from black to dark blue with shades of blue-green, green, amber, and gray in between. These color changes supposedly indicate your emotional state, with black indicating stress or anxiety and blue indicating happiness. But what the colors actually indicate are the degrees of warmth of your hands. They do this by means of sensitive thermotropic (responding to heat) crystals in or under the stone. Black = cold; blue = warm.

Because biofeedback training has been successful in helping people reduce symptoms in a number of stress-related diseases, such as high blood pressure and headaches, two investigators—Thomas H. Budzynski and Richard L. VandenBergh of the University of Colorado Medical Center—tried biofeedback-relaxation training with a twenty-year-old diabetic student who had been in the hospital eleven times with ketoacidosis (acid poisoning) during her first year in college. The doctors thought emotional upsets had contributed to her loss of diabetes control. Not only did learning "cultivated relaxation" help her lower her daily insulin from 85 units to 43, but she had no more hospitalizations for ketoacidosis and she felt that the technique helped her control her anxiety and tension levels and thereby stabilize her diabetes.

CHAPTER 8

Progressive Relaxation

Exercise therapists say that one of their greatest challenges is just getting people to know what a relaxed muscle feels like. Many of us have been so tense for so long that we consider muscular tension to be our natural state. These exercises are for those of you who can't tell a tense muscle from a relaxed one.

Progressive relaxation, or deep-muscle relaxation, as it's sometimes called, is a system of first tensing a part of the body and then untensing it in order to feel the difference and thereby become capable of making the transition from tension to relaxation yourself. It was developed over fifty years ago by a Chicago physician, Edmond Jacobson.

Dr. Jacobson based his method on laboratory experiments that proved that when your muscles are completely relaxed so are your mind and emotions. And what are relaxed muscles? They are muscles that are totally limp—that is, you are neither contracting (tightening) them nor holding them rigid.

Progressive relaxation is a very easy technique to learn, but it does require patience. It takes most people two or three weeks to learn the techniques if they practice half an hour a day, five days a week. You can hire a therapist who specializes in "Jacobsonian therapy," you can buy mail-order tapes to use at home (Check "Progressive Relaxation" on the Internet or on Amazon) or you can learn to do it yourself by reading our directions here.

The training program depends on (1) repetition—that is, *daily* practice—and (2) effortlessness, because the less conscious effort you bring to untensing the muscles, the more relaxation you attain. It's the old art dictum of "less is more."

Over and over in the learning sessions you experience the difference of sensation between extremely tense and extremely relaxed muscles until you can recognize the difference without any doubt or hesitation. Once you know exactly what your muscles are doing, you'll not only be able to control your tendency to tense up but you'll become aware when you're locking some part of yourself into a stiff, awkward posture that will eventually become your "natural position." In this way, you'll be able to avoid developing chronic tension in that set of muscles.

Now let's go through a practice session of progressive relaxation. You may want to have someone read this to you at first or, if you have a tape recorder, you may prefer to record it and listen to yourself telling you what to do. The value of this entire procedure is to plunge you into tension and then have the tension dissolve as you let go. You really only have to *think* about tightening a body part to engage the muscles, but in this practice session we're exaggerating to illustrate the contrast between tight and loose. Work slowly, holding each tension position for twenty to thirty seconds.

Sit in a high-backed chair or lie on your back on a carpeted floor or mat. Take a deep breath and hold it a moment. Breathe through your nostrils and from the abdomen, if you can. As you exhale slowly, try to let go of tension. Keep up a rhythmical pattern of breathing for a couple of minutes.

Direct your attention to your right hand. (If you are left-handed, start with your left hand and revise the following instructions accordingly.) Clench your fist tightly. Observe your forearm; see it become tight, too. Hold. Stretch your fingers out and allow yourself to relax again after twenty or thirty seconds of tension. Be aware of what is happening to your muscles, but don't be judgmental.

Make another tight fist with your right hand. Be aware of your muscles all the way up to your elbow. Hold. Let go slowly. Sense the difference between tenseness and relaxation.

Now, direct your attention to your left hand and make a tight fist. Notice how your arm feels. Hold. Slowly let go.

Next, push down on your chair or the floor with your right hand. Sense how your upper arm tightens. Hold. Relax and feel the flow of energy leaving. Now push with your left hand, hold, and then let go.

Hunch your shoulders so that you feel tension in your shoulders and the back of your neck. Make it extreme. Hold. Then float down. Let your shoulders fall. Sense the muscles tense and then feel them relax.

With your hands, arms, and shoulders relaxed, push the back of your head hard against the chair or the floor. Sense the tension in the back of the neck. Hold. Then relax and let your head float.

Now the chin. Tighten it. Clench your teeth. Hold. Then relax and allow your mouth to open a bit. Be slack-jawed.

Push your tongue against the roof of your mouth. Hard. Hold. Then allow it to flop down. Notice how it seems to get larger as it relaxes.

Tighten your eyes. The "purse-string" muscles go around them. Close the purse. Hold. Allow your eyes to relax slowly.

Frown. Make a deep, above-the-nose crease. Slowly relax. Do this particular exercise three times.

Next, raise your eyebrows all the way up. Hold until you get the feel, then lower.

The scalp muscle runs from the edge of the hair line to the back of the head. If you push your eyebrows, your ears, and the back of your head upward, you'll be contracting your scalp muscles. Hold. Now let down.

Tighten the muscles below your shoulders by arching your back. Hold. Then relax.

Next, tighten the abdomen—make it hard. Hold, then slowly let go.

The final step is to tighten your legs and feet. Stiffen your right leg. Hold. Relax it. Make your left leg rigid, hold, and then let the muscles smooth out. Study the feel of long, stretched-out, expanded leg muscles. Curl the toes of your right foot, making a "fist" of your foot. Hold. Then let go. Do the same with the left foot. Tighten, hold, release.

You will feel totally released from all tension—muscular or other-wise—at the end of your progressive-relaxation practice session. You will feel good all over. The more you practice, the deeper your relax-ation.

As you gain skill you can streamline your sessions and relax with-out tensing first. Just quickly check the different muscles in your mind.

The final stage of deep-muscle relaxation is to relax all of your body at the same time. Check for feedback from different muscles and relax any that feel tense. Finally, you should be able to relax all over in only twenty seconds or, if you get to be championship caliber, in only five seconds. Jacobson's goal with his patients was to teach them to relax muscles as quickly as they could contract them.

CHAPTER 9

Autogenic Training

- - - - - - - - - - - - - - - - -

Autogenics—the word means "self-generating"—is a tension-relieving method that involves repeating short, self-hypnotic sentences to yourself in order to influence your body to relax. For example, "My right arm is very heavy" is the first suggestion you give your body to help your muscles relax. You concentrate on creating, first, feelings of heaviness and then feelings of warmth. Feelings of heaviness indicate relaxed muscles and feelings of warmth indicate that blood vessels have dilated (relaxed). Once your right arm is heavy and warm, the body communicates this message to other muscles and you slip into a generalized total-body state of relaxation.

Autogenic training was perfected in Europe in the 1930s by a German doctor, J. H. Shultz, and has been widely known and used as a therapy there, and is now catching on in the United States. In Europe the training is usually given by physicians. Americans are being introduced to it through pain clinics and self-help books.

We're going to teach you the autogenic training formulas in stages, because that's the best way to learn them—in fact, the only way to learn them. We'll divide Dr. Shultz's original script into six parts: (1) heavy arms and legs, (2) warm arms and legs, (3) calm heartbeat, (4) regular breathing, (5) warm abdomen, and (6) cool forehead.

We recorded a cassette tape of the entire autogenic-relaxation script as presented here and used it ourselves over a period of several weeks and also tried the tape on several friends. We found that it works well for almost every accepting person whose mind is not closed to self-hypnosis.

In the beginning you are supposed to practice three times a day—after lunch and dinner and before going to bed. You can either lie down on a couch or bed with a pillow under your head and neck, assuming the yoga relaxation position, or sit in a high-backed straight chair.

Close your eyes, breathe deeply, and exhale slowly a few times to get general body relaxation, and then *slowly* repeat to yourself the following sentences. As you say each sentence, concentrate on that part of your body and feel it doing what you are telling it to do. Repeat each sentence four times.

STAGE 1: HEAVINESS
My right arm is heavy
My left arm is heavy
Both arms are heavy
My right leg is heavy
My left leg is heavy
Both legs are heavy

STAGE 2: WARMTH
My right arm is warm
My left arm is warm
Both arms are warm
My right leg is warm
My left leg is warm
Both legs are warm

STAGE 3: CALM HEARTBEAT
My heartbeat is calm and regular

STAGE 4: REGULAR BREATHING
My body breathes itself

STAGE 5: WARM ABDOMEN
My abdomen is warm

STAGE 6: COOL FOREHEAD
My forehead is cool

At the end of your practice sessions you have to bring yourself back to an active state, canceling or inactivating the training formulas by saying, "Arms firm, breathe deeply, open eyes." You have to be very careful not to forget this canceling sentence or you'll be trying to go about your regular activities with various parts of your body semihypnotized.

It may take you no time at all—only a session or two—to get through stages 1 and 2 and warm your arms and legs. And then again it may take you several weeks. We have to be so vague because it all depends on how suggestible you are. Some people, Barbara among them, have only to let a thought walk once across their minds and their bodies pick it up and go into action. Not surprisingly, therefore, it took Barbara only one session of autogenics to be able to warm her hands to the point of practically being able to fry eggs on them. June's suggestibility was initially much lower, but with practice she's increased her mind power amazingly.

Spend as much time as you need to on each stage in order to master it completely before going on and adding the next one. When you can go through the entire sequence of formulas from heavy arms to cool forehead in under five minutes, you can abbreviate the sequence into "My arms and legs are heavy and warm . . . heartbeat calm and regular . . . my body breathes itself . . . my abdomen is warm . . . my forehead is cool . . . ," plus the canceling formula, "Arms firm, breathe deeply, open eyes."

When you advance to this point, you can add additional autosuggestions directed specifically at helping you control diabetes or diabetes-related symptoms. Dr. Hannes Lindemann, author of *Relieve Tension the Autogenic Way*, suggests that a diabetic might say, "Pancreas flowingly warm," but we find that sentence not flowingly smooth (it's a translation from the German). Maybe you'd prefer some suggestion of your own devising, such as "Pancreas working calmly and perfectly" or "My blood sugar is normal."

We'd like to warn you not to get discouraged if you experience the slipping-back syndrome. That is, you may seem to deteriorate in your ability to respond to these self-commands, but with continued practice you will surge ahead again. Also, there is the possibility of what are known as "autogenic discharges" during the practice sessions. These are such things as muscle twitching, trembling, crying spells, and nausea. They're perfectly normal when unstressing, and meditators experience them, too. Just don't feel frightened if they should happen to you.

What we ourselves particularly like about the training is the total-body relaxation we can achieve with it. In fact, we both still use autogenic formulas for putting ourselves to sleep at night after a tension-filled day. June uses them for putting herself back to sleep if she wakes up in the wee hours with a reaction and has to get up and eat a snack.

CHAPTER 10

Meditation

Meditation comes out of Eastern mystical tradition. We're concerned here not with the complex, centuries-old religious teachings of Buddhism associated with meditation, but with meditation as a relaxation and calming technique. It's our impression that some doctors shy away from recommending it because of its religious implications. But to quote Eknath Easwaran, author of *The Mantra Handbook*, "Meditation is not a religion; it is a technique which enables us to realize for ourselves the unity of life within any of the world's great religious traditions, or even if we profess no religion at all."

Meditation is a generalized unstressing technique that releases you from your thinking machine, from that restless voice inside your head that never lets up on you except when you're asleep or unconscious—your "monkey mind." Thubten Chodrom, author of *Taming the Monkey Mind*, describes this simian sensibility thusly: "One of my teachers often compared our minds to monkeys': just as monkeys play with an object for a few moments and leave it in boredom and dissatisfaction to look for another thing to amuse them, so too do we run from thought to thought, emotion to emotion, place to place." (We Americans are particularly susceptible to monkey mindedness.)

What we particularly like about meditation is that if you carry it off, it gives you a wonderful respite from that problem you carry around in your thoughts all your waking hours—your diabetes. If you practice consistently, meditation can change not just your physiology but your entire life.

BUSY DOING NOTHING

The objective in all meditation is to control the attention. What you do is block out the outer world and submerge yourself in your own inner world. Each school of Buddhism, each branch of each school, even each yoga or Zen master seems to have a particular set of instructions for how to do this. Transcendental meditation (TM) is the meditative technique most of us have heard about, because it's been well publicized and advertised in the United States by its founder, Maharishi Mahesh Yogi. In TM, you restrict your attention by repeating a sound (mantra) over and over again while sitting with your eyes closed. TM is based on an East Indian form of Buddhism. In Zen, the Japanese form of Buddhism, you open up your attention by concentrating on your breathing.

We're going to discuss here only the beginning exercises for each of these two types of meditation. What we tell you may sound simplistic, but, believe us, only the explanation is simplistic. The process itself is extremely elusive and takes dedication to master. Until you've tried it, you can't realize how almost utterly impossible it is to harness your mind or turn it off for even a few seconds, let alone for half an hour. (You *can* do it, however.) Nor can you realize what a stunning relief it is from your normal state of awareness when you finally manage to do it, even briefly.

WHERE AND WHEN TO MEDITATE

Meditation should always be practiced in the same place, someplace where you will not be interrupted and where there is no noise. Finding this serene atmosphere is often the biggest challenge. June uses a small dining room that looks out onto the patio.

There are numerous traditional positions for meditation. The classic is full lotus. To do this, you sit on a small cushion on the floor, placing your right foot on your left thigh and your left foot on your right thigh. But half lotus (right foot on your left thigh or vice versa) and even just sitting on the edge of a chair are perfectly acceptable for beginners and for those who don't want to risk cutting off their circulation. Select the position that suits you best. If it's not too cold, purists suggest doing your meditation in bare feet. Removing your wristwatch is also recommended.

June finds it a good practice to meditate at the same time each day and looks forward to this time as free from stress. Early morning, on arising and before taking her insulin is the best time for her. (Meditating after eating is not recommended.) Before dinner is good, too, but before going to bed is not, as it may heighten your consciousness so much that you can't get to sleep.

Start with five minutes a day and gradually extend the time until you can handle as much as half an hour. A short meditation done daily is far preferable to a longer one done erratically. And if you have to change time or place occasionally, do so rather than eliminating that day's practice entirely. You need regular practice to create that oasis in your daily life where stress dare not visit you.

TRANSCENDENTAL MEDITATION

Let's begin with transcendental—mantra or sound—meditation and then go on to Zen—breathing—meditation. The first step is to choose your sound. The mantra is usually short, as short as a single syllable or two, and should have a melodious sound. The TMers say it should have no special significance, but in much Hindu yoga practice, the mantra is often an inspirational passage of several syllables or even words. Patricia Carrington, a Princeton University psychologist who uses meditation for mental therapy in her counseling practice, suggests that students in her program pick whichever of the following mantras sounds to them most pleasant and soothing: ah-nam, shi-rim, or ra-mah.

We ourselves like Diana Guthrie's idea of choosing a scripture to meditate upon. She uses "Be still, and know that I am God" (Psalms 46:10). Each time, as she repeats this verse, she makes it a shorter and shorter mantra by gradually eliminating words until she is down to the two words "Be still" and finally just "Be."

To do your mantra meditation, go to your chosen spot and take your chosen position. Take a few slow, deep breaths to quiet yourself, but not so deep that you become light-headed. Then close your eyes and start repeating your mantra slowly to yourself over and over again, breathing abdominally through your nose. As extraneous thoughts and images crowd into your mind, just let them flow through without allowing them to distract you from concentrating on your mantra. (When you are in this state, you cannot concentrate on any aspect of your diabetes.)

When you meditate it is something like placing yourself in an isolation chamber. And like the other unstressing techniques, it's virtually an impossibility to explain how to do it. In fact, some Indian teachers say that you don't "do" it. You create in yourself a state of nondoing and meditation happens spontaneously.

When you finish, stop repeating the mantra and sit, with your eyes still closed, for several more minutes. Rather than snapping yourself out of your meditative state, open your eyes, stretch the way you would when awakening from a nap, and then get up and resume your normal activities. You will feel refreshed and energized.

ZEN MEDITATION

Turning now to the Zen technique, how you sit is very important. As previously described, use the full- or half-lotus position, or sit on the forward part of a straight chair. Your spine should be straight, the small of your back concave (abdomen pushed out), and your chin pulled in. Keep your hands in your lap, turned up, with the left hand inside the right, unless you're left-handed; in that case, the right hand should be inside the left. Your thumbs should be lightly touching. Keep your eyes open, looking about three feet in front of you and downward, but unfocused. Begin by moving your torso in a wide circle, gradually narrowing the circle until you come to a stop at your natural center, where you will feel balanced and secure.

Now sit there and let your mind follow the movement of your breathing. Use abdominal breathing: in and out, in and out. Let other thoughts and images come but also let them go as you continue concentrating on your breathing. You can count one as you exhale if this helps, or one as you inhale and two as you exhale. You can even count your breathing all the way to ten, but no higher, as it would be distracting. Eventually you will get to the point where you can just sit and feel your breathing without counting. In fact, Zen teachers (roshis) refer to Zen practice as "just sitting."

MEDI-TEACHERS

Many meditators feel that for any form of meditation you should work under the direction of a teacher, because you need someone to answer your questions and help you with uncomfortable emotional and physical side effects that may appear as you are becoming unstressed, the same as with autogenics. Our suggestion for finding a teacher is to check with community and four-year colleges in your vicinity. Many offer courses in meditation, and the classes are sometimes held at the headquarters of yoga or Zen training centers. Meditation sessions with a Christian emphasis are offered by some churches. You can find announcements about these in your local newspaper.

11

Guided Imagery

· · · · · · · · · · · · · · · · · ·

Guided imagery, or visualization, as some therapists call it, is the act of forming images in your mind to calm yourself or to solve life's problems. This technique offers you two important benefits. First, it allows you to escape from your daily tensions into a tranquil haven; second, once there, through the eyes of an imaginary adviser, you are at last able to look at the big picture of the whole integrated mind-body-environment complex of your life and see what out-of-focus elements are responsible for increasing your tensions and/or causing your blood sugar to bounce around.

As a technique of self-therapy, guided imagery has very respected credentials among therapists and psychologists, and recent studies of the brain's hemispheres are helping scientists understand how guided imagery works.

The brain has two hemispheres. The left hemisphere controls the right side of the body; the right hemisphere controls the left side. The left hemisphere is the verbal, logical half. The right hemisphere is where your intuition and creativity abide. This side works not with words, but with pictures, with images. For calming yourself and solving your problems, one guided-imagery picture from the right hemisphere is worth a thousand words from the left.

As the name of the technique suggests, you need a guide to lead you out of your left hemisphere and into your right. Diana Guthrie is such an experienced guide for diabetics that we're going to take you on your first guided-imagery journey the way she does in her classes.

Get really comfortable. If you have something tight on, loosen it up. Close your eyes, because this is something between you and yourself. Now listen to my voice. Think through what I am saying.

First you see yourself inside a box. It looks as if there isn't any way for you to get out of the box. You feel very crunched, very enclosed. This box can sometimes represent your diabetes or your problems or your fears. You look up and you see a hand reaching down for you. That hand could be a family member or a friend or your heavenly Father.

You reach up and grab that hand. You're out of the box—into a beautiful field. There are trees nearby. There's a brook nearby. The sky is blue and the grass is very, very green and very, very comfortable. You can be by yourself or you can have others join you. But you're very happy and you're very, very peaceful. And you feel really good about yourself.

As you start to turn around, you notice that your box has become bigger. You begin to recognize that you can alter that box. You can put windows in it and you can put a door in it. You can come and go at will. You can rest in it. You can feel comfortable in it, recognizing that, yes, it's still there, but now you have some influence over what you can do with that box.

Okay, let's go inside the box and you can find out. You can imagine that you have two warm heat lamps over each hand and you begin to feel your hands get warmer and warmer. You almost think that you're at the beach and the sun is beating down on your hands and it's getting almost too warm. In fact, they're feeling sweaty, it's so warm, so warm. But you feel very peaceful and very comfortable and very relaxed.

So this has been a session of traveling that can make you feel more relaxed and more at peace. And now before you open up your eyes, you slowly count 1, 2, 3, 4, 5, and you are feeling happy and peaceful and very, very calm. And you open your eyes.

Diana then has the class stretch and "wake up" slowly, because, as she explains to them, their external blood vessels are probably dilated and their internal ones constricted. Getting up too rapidly might make them a little light-headed. She uses this exercise with people of all ages, even very young children.

Now we're going to introduce you to another guide, to someone who can individually help you, to a very wise adviser. It's a person who knows much more about you than we ever could. Here's how you go about meeting this adviser.

Think about a calm and beautiful place, a place where you have been contented and at ease. It could be in the mountains or beside the sea or a lake or a stream or in the desert or the woods, anywhere that you feel in harmony with yourself and the world.

Close your eyes and go there. Visualize yourself walking into this calming place. Hear the sounds, smell the aromas, touch the foliage or the sand or the grass, feel the warmth or the coolness. Experience it with body and mind. Sit down and rest for a while, enveloped by the peace.

Gradually become aware that you are not alone. There is someone sitting nearby. It is a person who is wise and kind, all-knowing, all-understanding, all-forgiving. Perhaps it's someone out of your past—your grandmother or grandfather, an aunt or uncle, a teacher or counselor. Or perhaps it's someone you've never met—and yet you know each other. You know you can rely on this person to help you.

You smile at your adviser. Your adviser smiles back. You talk for a while. You ask if you can have help in finding some answers. Your adviser says, "Of course."

You ask a question. Perhaps it's not the most important question of your life at this early stage of your relationship, but still it's an important question. Wait for the answer. Give your adviser time to think and respond. Your adviser *will* respond.

Continue to sit calmly and think about what you have been told, with all of its possible meanings.

When you feel you have truly understood the message, thank your adviser and embrace him or her warmly before you depart. Say that you look forward to returning and talking again soon.

As you leave your peaceful place, you feel joyful, fulfilled, healthy, loving, and that most nebulous and sought-after of conditions, happy.

Visit your peaceful place and your adviser until all your life questions are answered. You will discover what changes you need to make and you will have the courage and strength to make them.

Perhaps you have already figured out who this adviser really is: your own inner wisdom. After all, only you have the knowledge and insight to answer the important questions you're going to be asking about yourself and your life. With guided imagery you can open a wonderful new communication between your conscious and unconscious minds and solve many problems, including your diabetes problems, through your own creativity.

SOME TIME FOR YOURSELF

With all of these unstressing techniques, the most important, and hardest, part is taking the time to do them. Sometimes it doesn't matter so much which method you choose as much as that you get out from under your routines and pressures and demands while you're practicing whatever method you prefer.

Some quiet moments alone just doing five minutes of deep abdominal breathing (inhale for a count of four, hold for eight, exhale for eight) can help. So can good old-fashioned daydreaming. Let your mind roll on to whatever pleasant spot you like and picture yourself doing whatever pleasant activity you most enjoy. You have to learn how to escape from the demands of others and carve out time for yourself to do these therapies.

You must have heard by now the basic psychological truth that before you can love others you have to love yourself. There are other related truths for you as a diabetic to remember. You have to take in order to be able to give. You have to be selfish in order to be selfless. You have to help yourself in order to be the most help to others.

Massage

The *Keeping in Touch Newsletter* of the Scripps Whittier Education/ Support Groups reported on an article on massage benefits for diabetes that first appeared in the October 2000 issue of *Diabetes Interview*.

The benefits include:

Relaxation. Because diabetes management is stressful, the sedating effects of massage are particularly helpful. According to the report, blood sugar can drop as much as 40 mg/d during a massage.

Circulation Improvement. Circulation of the blood and lymph are improved by a massage. This allows insulin, oxygen, and other nutrients to reach the body's tissues more effectively.

Tendons, Ligaments, and Muscles. High blood sugars can cause a thickening of connective tissue that can cause uncomfortable and debilitating stiffness. Massage counters this effect by reaching muscles and connective tissue, directly resulting in greater mobility.

They recommend that even if you can't afford a professional session, you can learn to do simple techniques on your own feet, legs, neck, etc. A recommended book on the subject is *Massage: The Ultimate Illustrated Guide* by Clare Maxwell-Hudson, a long-time practitioner and leading authority on massage.

13

Sleep

. . . .

SLEEPLESS IN SEATTLE—AND EVERY OTHER TOWN

One thing you definitely don't *have* enough of is time. There are still only twenty-four hours in a day but the things you have to do keep multiplying. How are you going to fit them all in? You'll have to take the time from somewhere. Not from work. Work keeps demanding more of your time and you don't dare refuse, especially in time of unemployment. Not from your family. Your family is the most important part of your life and you'll regret it forever if you take time from them now. Then there's your diabetes. What a great consumer of time that is, what with all the testing and injecting or pill taking and all the stopping and thinking about it that you need to do. You can't take time from that. Where oh where can you find the time? Ah ha! There it is before your very (closed) eyes. Sleep. Eight hours or so just waiting to be diminished for more important things. And diminish it we do.

Richard Carlson, in his book *Don't Sweat the Small Stuff*, offers the suggestion to get up an hour earlier than the rest of your family, and in that way you can get a lot done. True. And think how much you could get done if you got up two hours earlier, or three? Many of us are starting to do that. As a result, more and more people are running around with what William Dement, M.D., calls our national nightmare: sleep deprivation. As founder of the Stanford University Sleep Disorders Center and the American Academy of Sleep Medicine, Dr. Dement knows whereof he speaks and he speaks it loudly and clearly and eloquently, as we heard when he appeared on a Commonwealth Club of San Francisco radio broadcast.

Dr. Dement believes that people are sleeping less because they don't put sleep first. Check yourself out. Is getting enough sleep a first priority? Would you turn down a tempting social engagement or an enticing work opportunity to get your sleep? How much sleep do you need? That's an individual thing, but for most of us it's around eight hours. Just as the song says, "Lucky, lucky, lucky me. I'm a lucky son-of-a-gun. I work eight hours, I sleep eight hours, that leaves eight hours for fun."

How do you know if you're not getting enough sleep and are building up a deficit. The way you feel is the giveaway. Dr. Dement says that sleep deprivation causes you to feel tired rather than sleepy. We have a friend who has a tendency to yawn widely in our faces. That could be a clue, too, unless it's just that we're boring.

If you're willing to put up with feeling tired most of the time then maybe being sleep deprived is no big thing. What's wrong with a little tiredness? There's a lot wrong. Dr. Dement says that if you're going around half asleep, "you're a walking or driving time bomb." The National Sleep Foundation reports that "Fatigue contributes to more than 100,000 highway crashes, causing 71,000 injuries and 1,500 deaths each year in the United States."

Dr. Dement calls a sleep-deprived brain "a stupid brain" that might direct you to do some stupid thing that causes damage to yourself or others. The last thing you need is a stupid brain when you have to use it to handle the complexities of diabetes!

And a dramatic reason for people with diabetes to get adequate sleep was reported at the sixty-first Scientific Session of the American Diabetes Association. In their study of the effects of sleep deprivation, Dr. Eve Van Cauter and her team of researchers of the University of Chicago found that if the subjects had only four hours of sleep for six consecutive nights, young healthy men had blood-test results that almost matched those of diabetics. Their ability to process sugar was reduced by 30 percent and there was a major drop in their insulin response. Along with that, they had elevated levels of cortisol (a stress hormone), which can lead to hypertension and memory impairment. Dr. Van Cauter said that the test results were more like those of sixty-year-old men than young, healthy men in their twenties and showed that chronic sleep deprivation had the same effect on insulin resistance as aging. The study suggests that sleep deprivation, which is becoming more and more common in industrialized nations, may contribute to the growing epidemic of type 2 diabetes we're now experiencing.

On a more positive note, with adequate sleep you flat-out have a better life, more *joie de vivre*. Your mood and energy level improve markedly, you can concentrate better, you're more productive, and you have a lessened tendency to be depressed. It could even be that if you're feeling depressed a lot of the time it may be more due to the absence of sleep than the presence of diabetes.

If you have a tendency to feel tired or sleepy in the mid-afternoon, it doesn't necessarily mean you're sleep deprived, because our bodies are programmed to get sleepy at that time of day (it happens to 90 percent of the population). In that case, you might take one of those "power naps" that some forward-thinking companies are encouraging their employees to do to improve efficiency. Of course, if you *are* sleep deprived then it makes sense to add some sleep time in the middle of the day to help pay back your deficit. But it's as was said in a report on power naps on the Earth and Sky website: "A nap can energize a sleep-deprived person the way a fast-food hamburger can energize you if you haven't eaten all day. But it's not healthy to live only on fast food, and naps can't substitute for longer periods of healthy sleep."

There are some rules of the napping game, as delineated by a world-class napper of our acquaintance, C. Steven Short.

Don't take off your clothes, except maybe your shoes.

Don't nap longer than twenty to twenty-five minutes. After that it becomes *sleeping* not napping and when you wake up you may find yourself groggy and grouchy rather than revitalized. A daytime sleep of a significant length may also interfere with your main sleep that night.

If you're not in the habit of napping, at first you may not find it easy to drop of into napland, but just lie there quietly with your eyes closed. You may surprise yourself by soon being able to turn a nap on like a spigot.

If we've convinced you to at least investigate to see if you're living with the handicap of a sleep deficit, you could start by reading Dr. William Dement's book *The Promise of Sleep: A Pioneer in Sleep Medicine Explores the Vital Connection Between Health and Happiness and a Good Night's Sleep.* In it, Dr. Dement teaches you how to "reclaim healthy sleep" in your own life. As one reviewer put it, "This book will put you to sleep—and that's a compliment."

You could also check into the website www.sleepquest.com. Dr. Dement is their chief scientific adviser and writes a column for them. Sleepquest will also help you to link up with other sleep-related sites.

WAKE-UP CALL

Although the majority of us need our eight hours, there are those who not only get by but thrive on much less. Psychologist Rosalind Cartwright of the sleep disorders center at Rush-Presbyterian-St. Luke's Medical Center in Chicago said, "There are natural-born short sleepers who are perfectly healthy with six or fewer hours." An old boyfriend of June's was one of those. He only slept about three hours a night his whole life. There were advantages to this, including having a lot more working time than his colleagues. This enabled him to get his Ph.D. in about half the time. If you're one of these short sleepers, you must be aware of the fact and don't try to change, no matter what Dr. Dement and other experts say.

CHAPTER 14

The Sound of Music /
The Sound of Silence

. . . .

MUSIC HATH CHARMS TO SOOTHE THE SAVAGE DIABETES

One person's music is another person's irritating, almost literally deafening noise. If your idea of music is hard rock pounding from a boom box or car stereo, then that's not exactly what we were thinking of as a passport to tranquility.

"Rock is any music you don't like." "If the music is too loud, you're too old." Okay. We'll accept those definitions from the other side of the generation gap. But think it over. How many aging rock stars do you see wearing hearing aids? How many fans have to keep pumping up the volume over the years to get the desired effect?

Another negative factor associated with rock music is that much of it has an anapestic beat (duh-duh-DUM, duh-duh-DUM), which is counter to our heartbeat and arterial rhythms and can cause immediate physical weakness along with other unpleasantries. "Music Doc" Nadia Lawrence, DMA, describes it as "angry"—working against the body's natural rhythms. "A steady diet of it," she says, "just feeds into a buildup of anger and frustration against the world."

"Balderdash!"—among stronger expletives—say passionate exponents of rock, citing numerous revered classical works that employ the same "destructive" beat. (Just because certain music is deemed "classical" doesn't mean it can't be irritating and upsetting.)

Discordant music, whether rock or classical, is also detrimental. As Diana Guthrie points out in her *Alternative and Complimentary Diabetes Care,* it "has been shown to cause cells, visualized by high-powered microscope, to shrivel, while pleasant music sustains or enhances the cells' shape."

Although pleasantness is in the ear of the listener, most would agree that music that is soothing and calming, causing the shackles of stress to drop away, would fit into that pleasant category. This is the kind of music used in hospitals and rest homes to create a peaceful atmosphere and to enhance the mood for those suffering with emotional disorders such as anxiety or depression. Many people find listening to early music (Medieval and Renaissance) particularly efficacious.

When you're feeling down and out and defeated over your diabetes or anything else, the right music (for you!) can buoy you up again.

Some music therapists think it can do more than that and do it more specifically. Nadia Lawrence, for example, is a strong believer in the healing powers of traditional Chinese music. Recently recorded music from China offers therapy based on the ancient concepts of the five elements (wood, fire, earth, metal, water) and yin-yang balance, as well as breathing and meditation techniques. She has tapes and CDs available that are recommended for various body parts and ailments, for example for people with diabetes she suggests the ulcer CD and other CDs in the health sets that are aimed at the spleen/stomach/pancreas organ system (earth elements in Chinese medicine). But she actually prefers to consult with the individual patient, asking questions to determine which music would be most appropriate and then give a "musical prescription" for it. As she says, "Diabetics, among others, may find symptomatic relief by taking a dose of the prescribed music every day. It is beautiful and inexpensive medicine without any side effects."

To explore the principles and possibilities of Chinese music therapy further and even hear brief samples of it, you can check out the Nadia Lawrence website at globalvisions.org/cl/lawr. You can also contact her by e-mail (nadiamusicdoc@juno.com) or by phone (in California 310-393-1951 or from other states 800-244-4541). Her mailing address is 513 Wilshire Blvd, PMB 359, Santa Monica, CA 90401 USA.

THE SOUND OF SILENCE

"Silence is a healing for all ailments."

—BABYLONIAN TALMUD

If they suddenly discovered that silence would cure diabetes we'd be no better off than we are now. Silence is one commodity in short—in fact almost nonexistent—supply in the modern world. What with lawn mowing and blowing, trucks rumbling and rattling, planes and helicopters roaring overhead, sirens shrieking, and dishwashers and vacuums whirring and clunking, noise pollution is rife and getting rifer every day. What does all that noise do to you? Apart from damaging your hearing, it can cause irritability, sleeplessness, indigestion and ulcers, stress, high blood pressure, and, some experts are beginning to believe, cardiovascular problems and an impaired immune system—the last thing a person with diabetes needs! Prolonged noise also makes people more angry and aggressive and hostile. What are you to do about all this? You can become an antinoise activist, but that's a long-range and probably ineffective solution to this all-pervasive problem. A better idea is to try to fit some silence into your own home, your own life. Parents talk about their children needing a daily "quiet time" and make an effort to give it to them. You should make an effort to give some to yourself (when all else fails, wear earplugs).

Since, outside of a padded cell, it's unlikely you'll ever be able to get total silence in this world, you should go for the more benign "white noise" advocated as a therapeutic focus for relaxation by Diana Guthrie. To her this includes "sounds of soothing music (see above), waterfalls, ocean waves, birds, or breezes." You can make your own white noises by doing things like putting a small splashing, self-perpetuating fountain on the table, hanging wind chimes outside your window, building a softly crackling fire in your fireplace, or petting your cat and listening to her purr.

Bertrand Russell said, "A happy life must be to a great extent a quiet life, for it is only in an atmosphere of quiet that joy can live." So as you go about making your life as quiet as possible, we can now move on to the living joy of a blithe spirit.

PART 3

A BLITHE SPIRIT

Many moons ago, at the American Diabetes Association's annual meeting in Los Angeles, a very unorthodox wonder drug for diabetics was introduced in a lecture to a luncheon gathering. This drug had only been tested anecdotally rather than in controlled studies with laboratory mice, and the two persons who developed and introduced it were neither scientists nor licensed professionals in the field of diabetes. Before the presentation was over, however, the physicians, nurses, dietitians, educators, and executives of the ADA were all partaking of this wonder drug themselves and giving every indication of wholeheartedly endorsing it as efficacious in a program of diabetes care. The drug was called Hug Therapy. The popular acceptance of this unorthodox drug encouraged us—for indeed, in case you haven't guessed it, we were its formulators—to return to our experiential laboratories and seek out more unorthodox diabetes therapies for health and happiness. We herewith present them to you. While none of these therapies has harmful side effects or interactions, they do potentiate one another for the better. We recommend that you add them all to your diabetes regimen. No prescription required. Guaranteed to bring about the third part of your diabetes total health and happiness triumvirate: a blithe spirit.

CHAPTER 15

Travel

. . . .

SERIOUS NOTE ON A HAPPY SUBJECT

Travel lecturer and filmmaker Burton Holmes said "To travel is to possess the world." On September 11, 2001, terrorists tried to take that world from us. Won't happen. Not to Americans, the most wanderlustful creatures on the face of the earth. We'll have to adapt to necessary changes in travel, but adapt we will as we continue to go about our business and pleasure around the country and around the world.

During this travel transition period, we'll have to keep our eyes and ears open to information on how to take care of our diabetes—and ourselves—in air travel. Regulations on carrying diabetes equipment and supplies onto planes is constantly changing and varies from country to country. You'll need to seek out the most up-to-date and accurate information. Along with that you'll need to have some help along the way if and when things go wrong.

* *Search the Internet.* Using a search engine like Google or Yahoo, enter "Flying with diabetes supplies and equipment." Click onto the latest ones and you'll see what the most current regulations

are. If you don't have a computer, borrow one or use the one in the library. It's worth making the effort. The Children with Diabetes website has a good summary of what the regulations are as of this writing. ➤ **DiabetiLink #13:** Flying with Diabetes Supplies (See p. 278)

- *Call your local ADA.* They should be able to tell you what the latest rules are and/or direct you to the most recent issue of *Diabetes Forecast* that contains them.

- *Have a good travel agent.* You're constantly bombarded with radio ads for finding travel bargain rates on the Internet. Be ye not deceived. You'll maybe (and maybe not) save a few dollars but lose a vital travel life support system. Your travel agent will be able to tell you what the current requirements are for carrying diabetes supplies onto airplanes as well as routes along your itinerary. If you have problems in the air or on the ground during your trip, you have someone to contact to straighten things out. You can't rely on what radio consumer advocate Clark Howard calls "customer no-service" of the airline you're flying. Often when you're having troubles with a flight or a ticket, so are a bunch of other people. You'll need someone who can cut through the red tape and leap over the lineup of other disgruntled travelers in a single bound. That super someone, as we know from personal experience, is your travel agent.

- *Insist on a real ticket.* Speaking of tickets, you want a real, live ticket that you can hold in your hand. Airlines may fight you on it and even give you inducements to accept an e-(for electronic) ticket. The major problem with one of these is if your flight is cancelled— as it so often happens these days—and you have a regular ticket, you can hotfoot it over to another airline that has a flight you want to fly on and a seat available for you; you hand them your ticket, they'll accept it and away you'll go. No ticket, no possibility.

- *Call before you leave.* On the day of your flight, you should call the airline before you leave for the airport to make sure the flight has not been cancelled (sometimes the passengers are the last to know) or the time has not been changed or the flight delayed.

With the new regulations, you have to be at the airport so far ahead of time that if there is a delay of any kind you'll begin to feel that you're a prisoner of the airport and wind up so exhausted that you won't enjoy the first few days of your vacation or you'll be unable to efficiently conduct the business you're traveling for.

* *Pack a lunch or dinner.* We've always advocated this, way before 9/11 problems. Airline food is notoriously unpleasant going-on-vile, non-nutritious, totally inappropriate for a diabetes diet, and seldom served when you need it Now it's often nonexistent as financially troubled airlines cut back on food costs, especially on shorter flights (two hours or less). The only problem with bringing on your own food is you'll have to endure the baleful, hungry stares of your fellow passengers. You must be strong. Think of your delicious meal as a medical necessity—after all, it is.

Now that we've considered the increasingly difficult logistics of commercial flying, today, it's time to explore the more positive aspects of travel. In the immortal words of Todd Beamer, "Let's roll."

ESCAPING THE DAILY GRIND

Several years ago June—whom we call the woman who has everything—developed another health problem: intense and incapacitating chronic headaches. These had nothing to do with her diabetes, but it took us five years of research and experimentation to find out what they did have to do with and how to cure them. While in the throes of those headaches she noticed a strange phenomenon. Any time she went on a vacation, the headaches disappeared instantly. It was truly remarkable. On plane flights, hardly had the wheels left the tarmac when *poof!* a headache that had been clamped to her skull for a week let go and floated away—and stayed away for the extent of the trip. Then, upon her return home, it reappeared.

Some of June's acquaintances offered the theory that because she didn't have headaches on vacations, she must not like her work. She was obviously drumming up headaches as an excuse to get away from it. This was absolutely untrue and we knew it. She loved her work at the Valley College Library and was never in her life a malingerer.

We developed another theory. It must be the foul and fetid air in Los Angeles that caused the headaches, since as soon as she got into the pressurized cabin of an airplane, where the air was different, her headaches left. We offered this theory to one of the many doctors she was seeing at the time to try to cure the headaches. This doctor, an expert in sinus problems, said that the air could possibly be the cause. Many of his patients, he said, were affected adversely by the smog. In desperation, June moved to the desert, where the air was clean, or at least cleaner.

That worked for a few months, but then the headaches came back. She then moved to Laguna Beach, California, to see if sea air made a difference. Same story as above.

At this time, a headache specialist finally discovered the *true cause* of June's headaches: TMJ (temporomandibular joint) syndrome. This is a malfunction of the jaw-hinge joint. When that joint is off-kilter, it sets off pain that can wind up in any part of the body—leg, back, head. Why would the TMJ pain be any different on a vacation than at home? When she was at home and at work—with all the built-in stresses and problems of those two locations—she unconsciously ground her teeth (day and night) and that set off the pain. On a vacation, away from those stresses, she didn't grind and didn't get the headaches. The headaches were cured by realigning her jaw by putting crowns on her back teeth. This was an expensive proposition that health insurance wouldn't pay for because it was a dental procedure, and dental insurance refused to pay because it was done to correct a medical problem. (That was almost enough to start her teeth grinding all over again!)

They always say that you can't leave your troubles behind when you go on a trip. They are wrong! We find you *can* leave them behind, and the farther you're away from them the better. You realize you can't do anything about your problems from this distance, so you finally put them out of your mind and decide just to relax and enjoy yourself. The stress-reduction techniques we described before are like mental mini-vacations. The real thing works even better.

Now, while you probably don't have TMJ syndrome, you *do* have diabetes; and literally getting away from your daily stresses can make your diabetes easier to control. Sometimes almost too easy. June has found that on a vacation when she's relaxed, her blood sugars start dropping hazardously and she either has to cut back on her insulin or eat more. This happens to her almost as quickly as getting rid of the headaches in the past.

IN TRAINING FOR TRAVEL

William F. Buckley once said that good training for the sport of yacht racing would be to stand in an ice-cold shower tearing up dollar bills. What with escalating costs the second part of that training session might work for travel as well.

But seriously, folks, for a successful trip some training is essential. The best training, of course, is a lifetime of travel experience. It's always sad to see people who save up their travel for when they retire, planning to take a "Really Big" trip then. (An inveterate traveler friend suggested that would be like abstaining from sex your whole life planning that when you retire you'll go out and have a real orgy.) More often than not, people who don't travel until retirement cut out on the trip early because they're not enjoying themselves since they're not in training, not used to the inevitable vicissitudes of travel.

So the first piece of advice is *travel now.* Don't wait. And certainly don't use your diabetes as an excuse to delay. Your diabetes is going to be a lifelong companion, so teach it early on to be a good travel companion.

Dry Run

If you haven't done much travel—especially after the advent of diabetes—before launching on a major excursion you should take a small weekend trip to someplace nearby. Pack all your diabetes supplies and any other health supplies you may use. (*Tip:* Get one of those plastic cosmetic bags with zippered compartments and a hook for hanging. These can be rolled up and tied for easy packing and unrolled and hung up on a shower curtain rail or towel rack. Mark all the compartments to indicate what's in each. When we travel together, we have one with compartments marked "June," "Barbara," "Mutual," and [the biggest one] "Diabetes.")

On your dry run, experiment with the comfort and wrinkleability of your wardrobe. See if you have everything you need to wear. And, just as important, see what items you can get along without. Build up your confidence about eating out three meals a day. Then, when the real trip comes, you know exactly how to pack and unpack and, most of all, to enjoy yourself.

Companion

Diabetes is a companion you can't travel without. All others are optional. As Hemingway said in *A Moveable Feast,* "Never travel with someone you don't love." We even know some devoted husbands and wives who can't travel together because each has diametrically opposite ideas of what a vacation should be. Test out your travel companion on that dry run just as carefully—or even more so—than your wardrobe.

Do you have the same rhythms of life? Are you both morning or evening people? Do you both like a tidy room or a messy one? And—this is vital—do you have a similar sense of humor, particularly an appreciation for the ridiculous?

You must also give your travel companion a crash course in diabetes so that he or she will be able to handle emergencies. See if the person can be relaxed about the situation. If someone looks terrified at the very thought of a diabetic emergency, shop for another companion. You also might shop for things that abort emergencies. For example, one friend of ours, Laura, almost lost her best travel companion when she passed out during a midnight hypoglycemia attack. The friend was so frightened that she refused to travel with Laura because it might happen again. Laura solved the problem by getting a Sleep Sentry (see p. 21) to wear in the night and beep her awake if her blood sugar started plummeting.

Insulin-takers should always stock plenty of blood-sugar–raising snacks as well as glucose tablets and one of the gels like Insta-Glucose or Glutose.

Footwork

An army may travel on its stomach, but tourists travel for the most part on their feet. That's why for an agreeable trip you need comfortable feet and legs in good muscle tone. Before your trip, get two pairs of comfortable walking (or running) shoes. Break them in with a gradually increasing walking program. Try to get up to three or four miles at once before you leave. Also be sure you do some of your walking in hilly areas and practice climbing lots of stairs. The right socks, too, are important. Dr. Peter Lodewick, author of *A Diabetic Doctor Looks at Diabetes,* recommends—and uses—Double Lay-R socks. He says "These socks have a thin, two-layer design that cuts down on friction and sweat buildup. The navy has found them effective in preventing blisters in their field marches, which include carrying a forty-pound pack for forty to fifty miles." You probably won't be doing that, but it's nice to know you could if you wanted to. These socks are available in sports and diabetic models. The diabetic ones have less nylon in the cuffs and are less restrictive. For more information you can call 1-800-392-8500 or check out the website at www.doublelay-r.com. For socks for heavier-duty outdoor activities such as hiking and backpacking, visit www.techspun.com. P.S. For years, cotton socks were what everyone was told to wear, but those days are gone. Cotton absorbs and holds moisture. Damp socks and feet are exactly what you *don't* need for travel, or anything else.

Airport

Whether your travel is foreign or domestic, you'll definitely spend a lot of time in airports these days, what with all the security checks and delayed and canceled flights. If you *really* want to train for travel, go out and spend twelve hours in a local airport. Bring along food enough for a couple of meals—or try to piece nutritious meals together from the airport eateries (real challenge, that one!). Practice sleeping on a bench or propped up in the corner of one. Learn to amuse yourself with crossword puzzles or a book or by chatting with other delayed travelers. Load your syringes and shoot in darkened restrooms. Develop your aplomb at taking blood sugars in public. Learn how to get into what marathon runner Frank Shorter calls his "travel mode," in which you stay relaxed and let nothing bother you. (As we keep emphasizing, stress shoots up your blood sugar faster than pecan pie!)

A GRAB BAG OF UNCONVENTIONAL TRAVEL RULES

You've probably read the basic travel rules for diabetics (take double supplies and a prescription for everything, keep supplies with you at all times, take two pairs of comfortable shoes, take diabetes I.D. in English and languages of countries visited, and so on) so often that you'll feel you need to take Dramamine if you hear them one more time. That's why we're digging deep into our collective travel reticule to try to come up with some slightly different but equally important rules for a happy, healthy, and successful trip.

We can't take credit for the first two rules. They were conceived by a nondiabetic foreign correspondent, which just goes to show that rules for a diabetic are often not that different from those for Everyperson.

Always Go to the Bathroom Whenever You Can

This means go when there's an opportunity—whether you really need to or not. In travel you never know when the opportunity will present itself again. In foreign travel this is particularly important. It's not that easy to find restrooms overseas. The *New York Times* Travel section once featured a whole article on how to find a restroom in Rome, thus acknowledging that it's a real challenge. Service stations overseas don't always have them and when they do, it's as it was with a friend of ours who stopped at an isolated French service station. He asked where the restroom was. The attendant fixed him with a gimlet eye and asked if he wanted to buy gas. When he said no, he didn't need any gas, the attendant firmly stated, "*Pas d'essence; pas de toilette* [No gas; no restroom]."

Even on home ground, though, this rule should be observed as a safety measure, especially in automobile travel. A psychologist friend told us her doctor brother maintains that in automobile accidents more damage is done by full bladders exploding on impact than by almost anything else. She won't let guests out the door to go home without first visiting the facilities.

Of course, for diabetics, back in the olden days of urine testing, there was a double reason for following the war correspondent's rule. But now, since the golden age of blood-glucose monitoring is here, you might add to this rule:

Always Test Your Blood Sugar Whenever You Can

When traveling, you may be going into different time zones and may be either more relaxed or more stressed. You may be more tired than usual. Your body has a lot of unfamiliar sensations and you may not pick up on your usual signals. June usually tests about twice as often when traveling since she wants to be able to catch a falling blood sugar before it gets too low or nip a rising one in the bud. Only by keeping your blood sugar in excellent control can you feel your best on a trip, and it's a shame to waste a trip by not feeling top-notch every minute.

If you're traveling by automobile and you're the driver, you should always test before getting behind the wheel, and every time you stop for a restroom break. It's just basic good sense for self-preservation and the preservation of others.

Never Take More Luggage than You Can Carry at a Dead Run for 150 Yards

Naturally, a war correspondent might have more reason to run than the average traveler, and for most of us, carrying a well-loaded travel purse or in-flight bag at a dead run for 150 yards might be more of a challenge than we'd care to take up. But the point is well taken. Don't take more luggage than you can carry yourself because you may be the only person around to do it (and you'd *never* want to leave part of your luggage unattended while you carry the other part). In fact, you really shouldn't let your luggage out of your sight, especially that part of it with your diabetes supplies. Just this year, two separate sets of friends traveling in Europe had their rental cars broken into at high noon while parked on busy streets. One was in Aix-en-Provence, the other in Genoa. They just left their cars for a little over an hour while they ate lunch. When they returned, they were picked clean, not even a road map left. The police could do nothing but commiserate and shrug—"It happens all the time." These people had to go out and find new clothes, toilet articles, and cameras. Suppose diabetes equipment and supplies had been stolen. Where in Genoa or Aix would you find another meter and strips and your kind of insulin or oral hypoglycemics? Unfortunately you aren't much safer from the brigands in the good old U-S-of-A, so always carry your bags with you. But we'll modify the rule to the extent that you don't *have* to carry them at a dead run. Incidentally, a divorced friend of ours—an avid traveler—who vowed never again to remarry, surprised us by suddenly doing just that. When we asked her why, she explained, "On trips, I needed someone to watch the luggage when I went to the bathroom."

ASSUME ANY PLANE YOU TAKE WILL BE LATE

The old adage, "If you've time to spare, go by air" has never been more true. Post-9/11 flights have become more and more unreliable in their take-off time. Flights are so irregular now that it is even said that most airlines have two schedules: the one they advertise and the actual one used by the airline personnel, which is almost invariably later.

This is significant for a diabetic in many ways. Meal times can be thrown off and your system can be calling for food when the airline is announcing another delay in take-off time. There may be no food available in the airport, or the airport is so crowded with other delayed-flight people that you can't get to it. If you must travel at a time when you will be needing a meal, to be on the safe side as we previously mentioned, you should bring plenty of appropriate food with you.

Delayed flights can cause an extreme stress response very detrimental to your blood sugar: as the adrenaline you're pumping signals your liver for fight or flight, it sends out the sugar to give you the energy to fight or flee. Since under the circumstances you can do neither, you just sit there with mounting blood sugar. The stress is lessened if you've taken our advice and already assumed the flight is going to be late. You haven't tried to make close connections with another flight because you know in advance you couldn't possibly arrive in time for one. You've probably even decided in advance to stay overnight and catch the continuing flight the next morning. Then if some miracle occurs and the flight *is* on time, you can consider it a thrilling surprise and a bonus to your trip.

Upgrade Whenever and However You Can

Most articles on travel try to tell you how to pinch pennies and find rock-bottom travel bargains. Often following this advice, you can wind up in uncomfortable situations (translation: flea bags and greasy spoons) that wear you out, spoil your trip, and run down your health. Don't get us wrong—we believe firmly in bargains, but what we like are *upgrade bargains.* These are arrangements whereby you can have something really nice, maybe even wonderful, for the price of something basic. There are more of these appearing every day as the competition for the tourist dollar increases. If you're a regular flyer, you undoubtedly already know about joining up with the various airlines for their frequent-flyer bonuses. Although it takes an awful lot of air miles to get a free ticket, upgrades to business or first class don't take nearly as many, and if you get yourself an airline credit card and put all your purchases on it, the points add up fast. (Warning: Always pay off your credit card balance every month, otherwise your only trip may be to debtor's prison.)

We've heard people question the value of business or first class for a diabetic who can't eat all that food and certainly can't drink all that alcohol. True. But you can stretch out and sleep in all that seat and arrive ten times more refreshed and ready for action than if you had been sardinized in the tourist section of a full plane. And, as for the food, true you can't eat it all, but you can eat what you want when you want it. When the flight attendants have just a few people in first and business class to take care of, they can cater to their individual needs. So although we'll seldom—if ever—pay the inflated prices for these higher classes, we'll comb newspapers and magazines to find all the special upgrading deals we can.

But it isn't just on airlines that you can get luxury for the price of basic. In major cities, the best hotels offer special weekend packages that work out to be much less than their weekday rates, when the hotel is full of business people. On these weekend specials they often throw in a few other goodies—like a meal in their restaurant and fruit in the room. Ask your travel agent about these specials and look through the travel section of major city newspapers. By the way, these weekend specials aren't just in this country. On a recent trip we found they were available in both Paris and London, making those two horrendously expensive cities only terribly expensive.

At resort destinations such as Santa Barbara, it often works the other way around. Weekends are when everyone wants to go there so the bargains are available in midweek.

YOUR DIABETIC PASSPORT

We mentioned that diabetes is a companion that you can't travel without. Happily it can turn out to be a boon companion.

The first thing to remember is to be totally accepting of your diabetes. Never hide it or act embarrassed about it. Since we're always upfront about June's diabetes, it has given us some pleasant adventures and allowed us to get acquainted with some wonderful people.

In *The Peripatetic Diabetic,* we reported how—when we were in Sri Lanka and visited a Buddhist temple in Mount Lavinia—a diabetic priest became so excited when he learned that June was diabetic that he went racing back to his quarters to get his "diabetes pills" to show her. He then gave us a wonderful personal tour of the temple.

One night in San Francisco we were dining at Trader Vic's. The room was dark, as Trader Vic's often tends to be. June didn't feel like trying to find the restroom to take her shot, so she just asked Barbara to discreetly give it to her in her arm. Later, when the maître d' came by to take the order, he said he had noticed what we were doing. He explained that he too was a diabetic and then spent time carefully going over the menu with us, explaining which dishes to avoid because they contained honey or sugar.

One of our favorite diabetic adventures took place in New York. Years ago when Barbara read the Dan Jenkins book *Semi-Tough,* she became intrigued by the repeated mention of bacon cheeseburgers at P. J. Clarke's (on Third Avenue at 55th Street). Her later study of New York City guidebooks revealed that P. J. Clarke's is supposed to be a hangout of the New York publishing and advertising set. Since that's the kind of people she likes to share atmosphere with, Barbara always insists on going there at least once every trip to New York, preferably the first night. (Yes, yes, we know that bacon cheeseburgers are hardly the kind of low-fat/high-fiber fare we generally recommend, but once a year doesn't hurt. *Remember the motto:* Moderation in all things—including moderation!)

On a recent trip to New York we arrived at the hotel around dinnertime. June wanted to take her insulin in the hotel before going to the restaurant—at P. J. Clarke's the restroom facilities are not exactly palatial and brilliantly lit. Since it was Friday, we knew there might be trouble getting a table. Barbara called for a reservation and became engaged in the following conversation with the maître d':

"Would you have a table for two in about fifteen minutes?"

"I think we could fit you in about then."

"Are you sure? You see, I have to know because I'm a diabetic and I'm taking my insulin right now and I have to be certain I can eat without too much delay." (Barbara often claims to be the diabetic. It takes any burden and embarrassment and *boredom* of having to say it off June, and since she isn't diabetic, she feels free about blurting it out. Other friends and family members of diabetics should try it.)

"Isn't that a coincidence?" said the voice on the line. "I just took my insulin, too. And, yes, you can be *sure* you'll get a table right away."

We weren't there two minutes before the genial maître d', whose name we later learned was James (for privacy we'll leave off the last name), escorted us to a table and made certain that we got attentive, friendly, and *fast* service. On our return to California we sent him a *Health-O-Gram* to encourage him to take good care of his diabetes. Then, as long as James worked there, every time we went to New York, we felt we had a home and a friend at P. J. Clarke's—all because of diabetes.

We've also met a lot of interesting, receptive people on planes. If June is going to take her injection at her seat—or Barbara is going to give it to her—we always explain to our seatmate what we're going to do and invite him or her to look away if it might be disturbing. This has been a great icebreaker. Almost every person we've encountered has a diabetic family member or friend and is interested in discussing the subject. One seatmate turned out to be a nurse, who criticized Barbara's injection technique because she didn't aspirate (pull back on the syringe to see if there was blood). This led to a lively exchange about whether or not aspiration is necessary. (We—and most diabetes nurse educators—contend that it isn't.)

These are just a few examples of the doors that the key of diabetes can open for you in travel. Don't keep it hidden in your purse or pocket, and you, too, can unlock many new and pleasant experiences.

Cautionary Note: Some people are allergic to even the most wonderful of wonder drugs. There are those who have an awful reaction to penicillin. There are those who get stomach distress from aspirin. And, sad for us to have to say, there are those few people who are allergic to travel. They just flat out don't like it, maybe even hate it. Although (as you may have gathered) we're not the slightest bit allergic to this wonder drug ourselves, we can understand their adverse reaction. Travel can be hard work. Travel can be frustrating. Travel can be exhausting. At times travel can wear down your health and upset your diabetes. For those of us for whom travel is as much of a life necessity as work, love, and oxygen, there's no problem at all with the trade-off. We hop to it without batting an eye. But if you're only traveling because someone else wants you to or because it's in style and everybody's doing it, you should stay at home and cultivate your garden or build a beautiful piece of furniture or do whatever it is you most like to do. Otherwise you're likely to wake up some night at 3:00 A.M. in a far-off somewhere, lying on a lumpy mattress, listening to someone trying to start a Vespa outside your window, your stomach burning with indigestion from the strange food, your feet aching from a day of treading the cobblestones, starting to feel the raspy beginnings of a sore throat, while you wonder if your blood sugar is low—or high—but you feel too tired to get up and test it. You start asking yourself, "How did I get into this?" We'd hate to have you say June and Barbara did it with their travel wonder-drug pushing. No, if you are definitely allergic to travel, then leave it on the shelf for others. After all, we still have three other wonder drugs for you.

CHAPTER 16

Pets

CREATURE COMFORT

Before Amy Miller, one of our diabetic employees, left the SugarFree Center to have her perfect baby, Andrew, she used to bring in her perfect beagle, Lester, every Wednesday afternoon. He spent his time in the patio off the reception area, where he was clearly visible to everyone who came in. Some of these people who came in were not in the greatest frame of mind because they had just been diagnosed diabetic and were scared and worried. On top of that, they may have been told to go out and learn how to stick their fingertips and take blood sugars and spend money they didn't want to spend on a machine they didn't want to buy to control a disease they didn't want to have. No, they weren't feeling too great. But if their eye chanced to fall on Lester, they usually smiled in spite of themselves. Often, after ascertaining that he was friendly, they would go out and talk to him and scratch him behind a floppy ear. You could tell they felt a lot better. We called Lester our pet therapist, deciding that in some cases he did patients more good than the most learned of diabetologists.

Although we accidentally discovered Lester's therapeutic benefits, our later reading and research revealed that pets truly do wonders for people's physical and mental well-being.

Dr. Elliot Joslin, in the original *Joslin's Manual,* gave a tribute to how much dogs have done for diabetics. He pointed out that not only did dogs help in the discovery of insulin but a dog is always ready to go for a walk with you. As you know from the exercise section, this is great for your diabetes control. Joslin also said that, best of all, a dog will never lap up some delicious dish that isn't on your diet and then proceed to tell you how fabulous it was—the way some people do.

PET RESCUE SERVICE

A dog can even save your life. At least one saved Candy Sangster's life. Candy was a longtime friend of ours at the SugarFree Center. One day she came in to tell us that her dog, Jet, had been nominated for the Ken-L Ration Dog Hero of the Year Award. She gave us a copy of the nomination write-up.

Dog's name:	Gridiron's Air Coryell (after Don Coryell, NFL Coach)
Nickname:	Jet
Breed:	Doberman pinscher
Gender:	Female
Age:	6 years
Weight:	75–80 pounds
Dog's favorite activities:	Riding in the van with her head hanging out the window; spending time with her owners
Date of heroic deed:	October 31, 1986
Owners:	George and Candy Sangster

Around dinner time on Halloween, Hazel Lavin heard a dog barking. It was Jet, the Doberman pinscher belonging to her next-door neighbors, George and Candy Sangster. Hazel looked out the window, saw nothing irregular, and returned to what she was doing. When the barking didn't stop, Hazel looked out the window again and saw Jet was in her front yard. She became worried. Jet wasn't the kind of dog who barked a lot. Stranger still, the Sangsters had trained Jet never to leave their yard without them. Hazel wondered how the dog had opened the gate without help. She then noticed that the Sangsters' front door was open and that the lights were on. She called Candy Sangster on the phone, letting it ring repeatedly. When no one answered, thinking something must be wrong, she called the emergency number, 911.

As soon as the paramedics arrived, Jet ran frantically between the driveway and the Sangsters' front door. She looked over her shoulder and waited for them. Hazel and the paramedics agreed that Jet seemed to be motioning them inside. The paramedics were a little apprehensive—Jet was, after all, a Doberman. But she wouldn't give up. Finally, with her eloquent dog body language, she convinced them to follow her into the house.

They found Candy Sangster on the living-room floor, unconscious. A diabetic, Candy had passed out earlier in the evening with severe hypoglycemia. As the paramedics worked feverishly to bring Candy around, Jet stood protectively by her side.

If not for Jet, the paramedics said, Candy would not have lived through the weekend, because her husband was out of town and not due back until Sunday, so no one would have been there to find her and call for help. Jet was the paws-down winner of the Ken-L Ration award!

FURRY BLOOD PRESSURE PILLS

But it isn't just dogs that work as wonder drugs. It's *all* pets. Cuddling a pet or even just watching one calms you down and lowers your blood pressure. A study at the University of Pennsylvania found that the survival rate for coronary patients was better for those with pets. Three deaths occurred among the fifty-three patients who were pet owners and eleven deaths among the thirty-nine who didn't own pets.

Dr. Karen Allen, a professor at the University of Buffalo, presented a fascinating study at a meeting of the American Psychosomatic Society. This study of one hundred women—half in their mid-twenties and the other half in their early seventies—showed that having a pet can lower your blood pressure. Half the women in each age group had a cat or dog that they loved very much and the other half had never even owned a pet. The women in each age group who had pets had lower blood pressure than those without pets. The blood pressure differences were the most dramatic in the older-woman group. In fact, elderly women with pets who had very little human companionship had blood pressure nearly as low as those of young women with lots of friends and family members.

A pet can also give an older person who lives alone or in an institutional setting a new leash on life. People in rest or convalescent homes who were in the depths of despair and wouldn't talk or interact with others often opened up in the presence of an animal. The Hillhaven Convalescent Hospital in Orange County, California, found that Mutty, who is part golden retriever, drew out an elderly man with Alzheimer's disease as no person could.

After the World Trade Center disaster, certified therapy dogs and their human partners were on the job accompanying family members walking the area around Ground Zero searching for lost loved ones and giving solace to those who realized that all hope was gone. Susan Urban, an associate director of counseling at the American Society for the Prevention of Cruelty to Animals, was quoted in the *New York Times,* saying "The dogs have worked the most wonders with men and boys, the tough type of people who don't necessarily know how to let go and show emotion." The emotionally and physically exhausted police and firemen had a particular need for the brief respite of a therapy-dog visit to the disaster site. Some pet therapists were even invited to attend memorial services and to visit fire stations that suffered the greatest losses.

The *Times* also reported praise of the dogs by Margaret Pepe, the disaster mental health officer for the American Red Cross: "I oversee 175 counselors, psychologists and social workers, and I wish they all had four feet," she said. "The dogs are incredibly effective, I'm jealous of the four-footed therapists and their ability to engage and relax people in a matter of minutes." (To learn about pet-therapy certification and registration programs check www.deltasociety.org and www.therapydogs.com on the Internet. There are also many local organizations. You may find information about these from veterinarians, hospitals, and nursing homes in your area.)

Janet Ruckert, a psychologist practicing in West Los Angeles, accidentally discovered the value of pet therapy when she had her cat, Clancy, in the office because she hadn't had the time before work to drop him off at the vet's for a defleaing. When a little girl with whom Dr. Ruckert had been making no headway started petting Clancy, she began to reveal her real feelings about her father, who had recently divorced her mother and moved away to start a new family.

Another time, Dr. Ruckert's rottweiler puppy, Lorelei, was in the office with her because she felt she was too young to be left at home alone. Lorelei trotted over and nudged a high-powered executive woman patient with whom Dr. Ruckert had been making little progress. When, at Lorelei's insistence, the patient started petting her, she was able to let down her barriers and express the softer side of her nature, her vulnerabilities, and her needs.

After these accidental encounters, Dr. Ruckert decided there was something to this and incorporated pets into certain of her therapy sessions. "Animals are natural therapists," she explains. "During a session not only does their presence allow a patient to express deep emotions and psychological needs more easily, but at home they are warm and sympathetic listeners." Dr. Ruckert is such a believer in the efficacy of pets that she's written a book entitled *The Four-Footed Therapist*. In it she describes what she calls "petcology"—the value of using the relationship of pets and people to improve everyday life.

A pet can be especially important to a diabetic child or teenager who may fear rejection because of being "different." There's nothing like unqualified, face-licking love to make you feel good about yourself. If you have no space for a cat or dog, have a cruel landlord who forbids them, or are allergic to animal fur or dander, a bird or a turtle or a tank of fish can provide calming comfort and—very important—something to love and care for and relate to. The living thing you love and care for doesn't even have to be an animal or bird or turtle or fish to help you with your physical and mental health. A poignant documentary film a few years back told of a lonely woman's love for a green bean plant she had growing in her window. When the plant died at the end of the film, as June put it in her mixed cliché way, "There wasn't a dry tear in the house."

So be it animal or vegetable (not mineral—pet rocks just won't cut it), get a pet. Your diabetes and your life will be better with one or more of these wonder drugs.

PET'S EYE VIEW

When we were publishing *The Diabetic Reader,* we always worked very hard on it so it was a little disconcerting when people wrote to say something like, "I just love Mary's column" or "Mary's column is my favorite part of your publication." In case you aren't familiar with Mary, she is Mary, Queen of Scottish Folds, the nation's premier feline diabetes journalist. Her column, "Animal Magnetism," appeared in each issue of the *Reader.* Here, for your delectation, are a few of her more popular columns, ➤**DiabetiLink #14:** The Best of Mary (p. 279) Note: if you find these columns your favorite part of the book, please don't write us to say so.

CHAPTER 17

Laughter

ACCENTUATING THE POSITIVE

We once received what could loosely be described as a fan letter from a reader of our book *The Peripatetic Diabetic*. The letter ended with, "I'm sorry, but I just don't find diabetes as much fun as you two seem to." We thought about that one for a while and then Barbara was assigned to write the response. (Since she doesn't have diabetes, she finds it a mite more fun than June does.)

Barbara wrote our correspondent that we feel that diabetics are well aware of the dismals of the disease. There's no need to have those dismals driven home to them in books and lectures. They have to live with them every day of their lives.

We feel it's our job to help diabetics look on the bright side and find humor and fun and laughter wherever they can, even in the diabetic state and its therapies. A humorist once said, "Just because I laugh at life doesn't mean I don't take it seriously." Just because we laugh at diabetes from time to time doesn't mean we don't take it seriously, and it certainly doesn't mean we don't want *you* to take it seriously. We just want you to keep your sense of humor alive because it's virtually impossible to have a humorous attitude toward something and at the same time to feel angry and resentful toward it.

Psychologist Dr. David Bresler of the UCLA Pain Control Unit says that he always wishes he could check a patient's serum fun level because those patients with a high serum fun level have a much better prognosis for recovery. "We want to make sure our patients have enough fun to break their negative life attitudes," he says.

One of the reasons laughter is such an effective diabetes therapy is that it's a great stress reducer. As Dr. Raymond Moody pointed out in his book *Laugh after Laugh: The Healing Power of Humor,* when you laugh you briefly lose muscle tone. All the tense muscles of the body are relaxed and you have what the British philosopher Herbert Spencer called "a discharge of nervous excitement." Dr. Moody reported that one physician friend found he could cure tension headaches simply by getting patients to laugh at him. Another physician found that all his very healthy elderly patients had one thing in common—a good sense of humor. All in all, Dr. Moody said, he had "encountered a surprising number of instances in which, to all appearances, patients have laughed themselves back to health, or at least have used their sense of humor as a very positive adaptive response to their illness."

Laughter, according to the late Norman Cousins, former editor of the *Saturday Review,* is a kind of "internal jogging" that can be even more health restoring than the external kind. Cousins was, in fact, living proof of the healing power of laughter.

He was lying in a hospital bed in agony, suffering from a collagen disease (a disease of the body's connective tissues) that a whole battery of experts couldn't cure. One day Cousins accidentally saw a letter his doctor had written to a mutual friend. In it appeared the sentence, "I'm afraid we're going to lose Norman." That did it. He decided it was time for him to get involved in his own case.

Since he knew that negative emotional states can make a person susceptible to illness, he reasoned that positive emotion might help bring about recovery. And what, he thought, is more positive than a good, straightforward, uncomplicated belly laugh? Cousins arranged to have videotapes of old *Candid Camera* TV shows played, and lo, after an hour of laughter he found his pain had diminished to such an extent that he could get a good night's sleep. When doctors performed tests on him after one of these laugh sessions, they found that the inflammation in his tissues had lessened.

Another aspect of Cousins' self-therapy that must have done much toward activating his joy gland and increasing his serum fun level was checking out of the hospital, with his doctor's approval, and into a luxury hotel. Not only was the cost considerably lower at the hotel (which contributes a lot to one's good spirits) but the food was more appetizing and the service just as attentive.

The end of the Cousins story was a happy one. He lived to tell the tale of his illness and unusual therapy in the *New England Journal of Medicine* and in the book *Anatomy of an Illness*. He went on to give guest lectures at the UCLA School of Medicine.

Now it's true that Cousins was also taking large doses of vitamin C, and his cure may have been brought about by that, or maybe it was just a matter of nature taking its course and he would have recovered no matter what he did. Still, deep down in our funny bones, we feel that laughter had a lot to do with it. We also feel that if you increase your own personal supply of this wonder drug it can't help but do good things for your health and your diabetes.

The big question, then, is where do you get a steady supply?

ELIMINATE THE NEGATIVE PEOPLE

Negative people are worse for diabetics than positive urine tests. As the French existentialist Jean-Paul Sartre said, "Hell is—other people!" But that's only half of it. Heaven can also be other people. You just have to find the right people, the positive people, the ones who fill you with joy and laughter rather than gloom and doom.

We have a term for these negative sorts—prana suckers. *Prana* is the Sanskrit word for life force, and after you've been with these people for a while you feel as if they've sucked the life force right out of you the way a vampire sucks blood. You feel totally drained.

One tendency of prana suckers is to be blemish finders. This means they only have eyes for flaws. If you take blemish finders into a room full of beautiful art objects except for one ugly little dirty jar off in a corner, they will ignore all the beauty and, scowling with disgust, say, "Would you just look at that ugly little dirty jar!" Even if you have a wonderful life full of activity, work, and people you love, there are bound to be some blemish finders who will focus on and tsk over your one flawed aspect—your diabetes—never mentioning all the reasons you have for happiness.

Prana suckers also seem to be full of what psychologists call negative expectations. They always know the worst is likely to happen—in fact, it definitely *will* happen—and they love to sit around with you and flip through their catalog of potential disasters. For diabetics, there are plenty of potential (yet avoidable) disasters that a person can dwell on if so inclined. And just as it's important not to dwell on them yourself, it's important not to hang around with people who want to dwell on them for you.

We're sorry to have to say it, but even doctors can be prana suckers. June's original doctor was a good example of this. He followed up the diagnosis in this delightful way: "Everything about your life is going to have to change. No smoking. No drinking. You have to watch everything—and I mean everything—you eat from now on. Take this diet sheet. If you don't follow this plan to the letter, you can go blind; you can get gangrene of the feet and have an amputation; and you can get kidney failure and die."

June's headache specialist, on the other hand, was exactly the opposite kind of doctor. His sense of humor was always operative. He was invariably hopeful and positive and, above all, he loved his work. We once saw him at a conference, eyes shining with excitement, describing "the fun and reward of helping a patient." *That's* the kind of doctor you should seek and find.

Sometimes, unfortunately, the negative people are family members and it's pretty hard to avoid them. But remember, negative people are like stress: it's not so much the people themselves as your reaction to them. You've got to keep their negativism from getting to you. You've got to learn to laugh them off.

Another approach is to look for the positives in negative people. No one is *all* bad and if you seek things to appreciate in negative people you shall surely find them. And as they bask in the glow of your appreciation, it may put them one step on the road to recovery from negativism. It's worth a try.

HOW NOT TO BE YOUR OWN WORST ENEMY

Sometimes you may find yourself falling into a slough of despond where you, yourself, become a prana sucker, where negativism reigns and no laughter abounds. When this happens the cause is often the horrifying "What if" syndrome. This works by making you imagine that something dreaded and feared will happen: What if I develop complications? What if I can't have children? What if my spouse can't stand my having diabetes and divorces me? What if I have an insulin reaction on the job and make a fool out of myself and my boss loses confidence in me and takes away all my responsibility and I never get another promotion and wind up getting laid off? You then take these imaginary happenings and proceed to fester and fret and worry yourself into a frenzy over this. This is totally counterproductive to enjoying life. Worry—especially worry over events that most likely will never happen—is a total waste of time and stomach acid. But what if (!) you intellectually know that, but you can't help yourself? These "what if" worries keep cropping up and clouding your life so the sunshine of good times can't get through. Can anything be done about it? Yes. You can pick up your lance, charge off, and start . . .

SLAYING THE WORRY DRAGONS

In her book *Making It Through the Night,* Marilyn Shroyer suggests a worrying self-defense technique. Set aside thirty minutes each day to worry, and then stop. During your designated worry time, you should make a worry list. Then rewrite this list in order of importance. Next, ask yourself what, if anything, you can do to change each situation. Calling upon all your knowledge and wisdom and information and experience, write out possible solutions. If you find there's nothing you can do about something on the list, scratch it off the list and forget about it.

Writing out all your worries is a good way to discover how unrealistic and unlikely most of your worries are and for working out ways to handle the worries (if any) that are valid and fixable.

Now that's the good, logical, left-brain approach for those of you whose minds work that way, but for right brainers—the artists rather than the scientists—here's another equally effective approach. In Carefree, Arizona, a man named Gregg Warren says he can free you from all your cares and worries for a mere $5. You write all your worries on a piece of paper and send them to him. He burns them, jumps into his plane, flies up two or three thousand feet over Carefree, and scatters your worries away.

This is not as nutty as it sounds. Once on a trip to Thailand, Gregg Warren met some Buddhists who burned things to get rid of their worries. They felt that thoughts are really things. And if the thoughts become worries, they must be released back into the universe as quickly as possible—otherwise they become suffering. We have a way to save you $5. Just send your worries to us c/o our publisher, fax them to 818-786-7359, or e-mail Prana2@earthlink.net. At no charge, we'll burn them and scatter the ashes into the Pacific (remember that means "peaceful") off the Stearns Wharf Pier in Santa Barbara. We'll love the excuse to go there, since it's one of our favorite places on earth. Ecological note: No need to worry about our contaminating the ocean or air with the trouble-eradication process. Once we burn them up, the ashes are so minuscule as to be virtually nonexistent—just as we hope your troubles will be.

COURTING THE "WELL AT LEAST" SYNDROME

You should always try to look for the positives lurking in every negative situation. Here's a technique for doing that. Barbara, who is almost pathologically positive and chronically optimistic discovered it. Here's how it works. She recently took her car in to have the coolant topped off because the air conditioner wasn't working too well. The mechanic started probing around the car's innards and found that not only did the coolant need to be drained and refilled, but every belt and hose in the car had to be replaced as well as the brake rotors and timing tensor (whatever that is!), plus a leaking brake master cylinder needed fixing. As she walked away after paying a bill of $809.45, she was heard to say, "Well at least I didn't need a lube and oil change."

To put this into diabetes terms, not long ago, June, after consuming a mystery dinner at a friend's house, found that she had a 200+ blood sugar. Instead of ranting and raving and accusing herself of doing something stupid as is her usual wont, she stopped and thought and applied the "Well at Least Syndrome" to the situation. "Well at least I don't have to waste time fixing and eating a bedtime snack." So you see, even an old dog with thirty-six years of diabetes can learn new tricks.

Another similar trick is, when you're experiencing a negative event, to follow author Catherine Ponder's advice: "When something bad happens to you, look at it and say, 'What good can come out of this situation?' because there are showers of blessings in every situation." Seeming disasters can turn out to be blessings with the right attitude. As the Buddhist philosopher said, "The barn has burned down, so now we can see the moon."

But what possible "showers of blessings" are there in having diabetes? Well, for openers we know many people who found their life's career through diabetes. We marvel at the number of diabetes health professionals (doctors, nurses, dietitians, etc.) who entered the field as a result of their own or a family member's diabetes.

Recently we read Jeff Weinstein's profile of superchef Wolfgang Puck in *Los Angeles Magazine*. The biographical information on Jeff read, "Weinstein has been fascinated with food his whole life." And they quoted him, "I've read cookbooks since I was a boy and there isn't a food that I'm not interested in learning about. If you say 'Tell me everything about oranges,' I can. Or apples. Or endive." Weinstein, who has been a restaurant reviewer for nearly twenty-five years, mostly for the *Village Voice,* is writing a book about hunger and pleasure. He says, "It's about being a diabetic and being obsessed with food, about how the two coincide. When you take insulin, it makes you hungry in the way a starving person is hungry—and that kind of hunger has always made me intensely focused on what I'm eating. It's the reason I've learned so much about food."

We've even known people who found their own true love through diabetes. In *Diabetes Forecast* magazine we read about one woman who was diagnosed diabetic just after graduating from high school. She was very shy and felt alone with her diabetes. In her loneliness she wrote to the Making Friends column in the *Forecast.* Among the many letters she received was one from a young Canadian man who was around her age and had been diagnosed at about the same time. They became instant friends and encouraged each other to not let diabetes get them down. After corresponding for three years she decided she should meet him and took a plane (her first plane trip ever) to visit him. They both knew immediately that they were made for each other. But they lived thousands of miles apart. He couldn't leave Canada, so the decision was hers to make. After much soul-searching, she quit her job, left her extensive family in the south, married her true love, and moved up to Canada, where they are living happily ever after.

Another love story—business success story—concerns Steve Yeager, the inventor of the Medicool (the case that keeps insulin cool). When his sister Suellen was diagnosed with diabetes, he created his invention and started his company in great part to help his sister and give her something to do to take her mind off her diabetes problems. She often worked with him at conferences and trade shows. At one such show there was a man who owned a medical products company at the neighboring booth. He and Suellen started talking during lulls when people attending the conference were at meetings. He asked her out to dinner that night, and they kept running into each other at one medical conference after another. Their common interests and friendship grew into love and now, they, too, are married and living happily ever after with diabetes as the matchmaker.

COINS IN THE BANK OF LIFE

Barbara has a theory that she admits most people consider the height of nuttiness. It goes this way: when something bad happens to you, it means you're putting a coin in the bank of life. And some time down the road, you'll be able to make a big withdrawal of all the coins—plus interest—that you've put in. Only now they have metamorphosed into coins of happiness. Try it. It may help you put a new, cheerier face on your troubles. At least it can't hurt.

WAKING UP YOUR DREAMS

And then there are your hopes and dreams. Often you have to delay your gratification of these until you get through a work project or finish a college degree or some such, but some people delay their gratification forever. They deny their dreams until it's too late to realize them. June has always had tendencies toward delaying gratification, but she's doing better at fighting those tendencies these days. Since she's one-quarter Dutch, her biggest dream always was to go on a bike tour of Holland. Finally, one summer several years ago, she delayed it no longer. And now, with her memory bank full of that trip, she's smiling all the way to the fulfillment of her next dream.

At the end of Amy Tan's children's book, *The Moon Lady*, the little girl heroine says, "And I knew what the best wishes were: those I could make come true myself." Those will be your best wishes and hopes and dreams, too.

A while back we received a letter from a young woman with whom we'd been corresponding. She is an artist whose dream was to write and illustrate a children's book. She happily reported that her dream had finally come true. She's finished her book, and she's positive it's going to be published soon. She wrote, "I do not love this disease, but it has been a force that has led me to do many things with great motivation, including public speaking. Living with diabetes has enabled me to reach one of my dreams because many years ago I accepted the diabetes within me and moved on to become all I can be."

Just as everything about your diabetes is very personal, so will your own particular dreams be personal. You may want to travel to some exotic place; you may want to take up a new activity like skiing or horseback riding or painting or studying music or even becoming an expert ballroom dancer as Betty Marks did. Betty is the author of several diabetes cookbooks and a literary agent by profession. All her life she pushed her clients along the road to their dreams. But after being diagnosed with diabetes and having a bout with cancer, she finally decided it was time to realize her own dream and to allow the luxury of indulging herself. She says, "Dancing has taught me how to focus, given me a greater sense of self-esteem, taught me to be self-reliant and yet work closely with a partner. But the greatest reward is that I'm smiling all the time." Betty, we might add, now has dozens of trophies and medals for competitive ballroom dancing.

Whatever you do, don't deny yourself your dreams because you're afraid your diabetes might cause some awkward problems. If you believe you can't do something you dream of because you have diabetes, think about Judith Oehler-Giarrantana. She's a nurse and rehabilitation specialist. She's also a blind diabetic. But she didn't let that stop her from becoming the first blind person to complete a rigorous Wilderness Survival course. Try on this quote from her for inspirational size:

The boat was completely open—no kitchen, bunks, or head (which meant testing urine over the side of the boat.) The first night I didn't do a urine test; it was difficult enough to learn to brush our teeth and take care of toilet needs over the side of the boat. The next day, however, I was comfortable enough to ask others to assist me.

And this:

The most difficult exercise was the split log. I had to cross two logs, suspended end to end twenty feet in the air, with a four-foot gap in the middle. I crept across, hanging on to a rope with an instructor verbally guiding me. When I got to the gap, I crouched down and stretched one foot across it. I had difficulty locating the other log with my foot so I returned to the crouched position to rest. The second time I was successful! After I had finished, one of the instructors told me that was the one exercise they had felt could not be completed by a blind person.

As she summed it up, "Outward Bound reaffirmed for me the necessity of taking meaningful risks in order to reach my full potential." We'll bet that her accomplishment gave her a big smile of personal satisfaction.

THE ULTIMATE CHALLENGE

So keep an optimistic attitude. Have all the good times you can, and you'll find you have the power to beat that old devil, chronic sorrow, and realize your dreams despite health limitations.

Bob Massie, an Episcopal minister and former candidate for lieutenant governor in Massachusetts, says that his life, which has been defined by the adversity of his hemophilia (chronicled in his parents' book, *Journey*) prepared him for that political race. Bob, who had to endure excruciatingly painful bleeding joints, underwent 497 transfusions from the time he was six until he was twelve. He had to use leg braces and a wheelchair. Eventually he proved wrong all the doctors who told him he would never walk again. His vigor on the campaign trail belied the hardships he has known. He is now HIV positive as a result of his many transfusions; nevertheless he keeps moving on toward his goals and dreams. "You cannot escape pain," he says. "Life is painful. There is loneliness, anxiety, and fear . . . fear of rejection, fear of deprivation, fear of death. Learning to cope with these fears and living a life of joy in the midst of all that is a great challenge."

We know you can accept that challenge.

THE GREAT PRETENDER

You may think this talk about laughter and smiles and how thera-peutic they are is all very well, but what if you don't feel full of fun and optimism with the specter of diabetes continually floating around in your subconscious? Well, then, what you do is just *pretend* you're a happy person.

Kurt Vonnegut had as the moral of his book *Mother Night,* "We are what we pretend to be, so we must be careful about what we pre-tend to be." Mark that well. Pretend to be a miserable, down-feeling, hopelessly sick person with your joy gland in worse shape than your pancreas and that's what you'll be. Act like a healthy, hopeful, vital person and *that's* what you'll be.

The homely philosopher Josh Billings, said "Laffing iz the sensa-tion of pheeling good all over, and showing it principally in one spot." With a little pretending it can work the other way around. You can "laff" even when you don't "pheel" so great and it can actually make you "pheel good all over." This is the premise of what Ajay Singh, writing in the *Los Angeles Times,* calls "a curious new phe-nomenon . . . dedicated to laughing for happier, healthier, and fuller lives." People gather together in public places or apartments for the sole purpose of "surrendering to uninhibited laughter." Sometimes there is a leader like San Francisco's "certified laugh leader," Kim Corbin, to put them though their laugh paces from "lion laughter" to "chicken skip laughter" to "silent laughter" to who knows what kind of laughter they'll come up with next. This therapeutic laugh-ing movement, which was started in India by Dr. Mandan Kataria, the so-called "guru of giggling," has grown to over one thousand laughing clubs in India and is beginning to snicker its way across the world. In 1998, when Dr. Kataria staged a World Laughter day at the Bombay race track, over ten thousand participants showed up for the mass chuckling, tittering, giggling, and guffawing celebration.

Aside from making you "pheel good all over," what does this staged laughter do for you? Try these purported benefits: it helps you lose your inhibitions and increase self-confidence; lowers blood pressure; releases pain-killing endorphins and produces anti-inflammatory agents that can reduce back pain and arthritis; alleviates migraines, exercises facial muscles for a more youthful appearance; makes you more mentally alert; lowers stress and relaxes muscles; and just plain delivers you from grouchiness, turning you into a more pleasant person to be around. (They don't mention helping control your diabetes as a benefit, but we think it can't hurt.)

If laughing only does half—or even a quarter—of the above, it's worth trying. You can start in the privacy of your own home and graduate to a group. You can find more information on the Web under the headings "laughing clubs" and "therapeutic humor" or check into the website www.worldlaughtertour.com. This international clearinghouse for information, ideas, and news about therapeutic laughter and laughter clubs was founded by Steve Wilson, M.A., CSP, and Karyn Buxman, CSP, CPAE. Their motto: "Together we can lead the world to health, happiness, and peace through laughter."

You might also check out a video of the movie *Patch Adams,* about a doctor who uses humor as therapy, and look for *The Laughing Club of India,* a documentary by the acclaimed Indian filmmaker Mira Nair.

Now to help you get started with your new happy attitude, we'll try to get you laughing with a story from the Prohibition era. It seems there was this drinking gentleman whose regular bootlegger was put out of commission by Elliot Ness's boys. The gentleman quickly found himself another bootlegger, but this bootlegger's product was a little strange-tasting. Since he'd heard stories of people being made sick, or worse, by bootleg whiskey, he decided to be on the safe side by sending it to a laboratory for analysis.

The report came back. "Dear Sir," it read. "We're sorry to have to tell you this, but your horse has diabetes."

CHAPTER 18

Hugs

· ·

A CALL TO ARMS

If laughter seems to be an unusual diabetes therapy, this one may strike you as downright outlandish, so we'd better give you a little of the background and scientific rationale of this wonder drug. Its discovery came about when Barbara, who was then a college librarian, read an article in a library publication that told of an experiment at Purdue University. The library workers were instructed to "accidentally" touch the hands of certain students as they were checking out books to them. The touch was to be so brief and light that the student might not even be consciously aware that it was happening.

Then members of the psychology department, lurking outside the library, would stop the students and interview them. It turned out that the students who had been touched had much warmer, more positive feelings toward the library, toward themselves, and toward life in general than those who hadn't been touched. Why was this so?

Well, as family therapist Helen Colton, author of *The Joy of Touching*, explains, "Our need to be touched, caressed, and cuddled is as basic as our need for food. . . . Without it we get a kind of malnutrition of the spirit."

As you must have noticed, our culture is not big on touching the way Latin and Mediterranean cultures are, so a lot of us are walking around with malnutrition of the spirit. These Purdue University students had for once had their touching needs met, and it was an almost instantaneous change from malnourished to nourished.

Barbara mused on this touching experiment and decided it was just what both the library and the students needed. We could combine great public relations for the library with improved mental health for students—something they especially needed in this era of lowered expectations when there might be no jobs waiting for them on graduation.

She announced to the staff of the checkout desks what she expected them to do. Uptight puritan types that they were, they flatly refused to give students a subtle nourishing touch along with their books. "All right," said Barbara like the Little Red Hen, "then *I* will." But though she had every opportunity to touch when helping students with the periodical indexes, she couldn't bring herself to do it. It somehow seemed sneaky and furtive to be "accidentally" brushing against students' hands. The good idea appeared to die a-borning.

But then, about this time, we were talking to Dr. David Bresler of the UCLA Pain Control Unit in conjunction with our headache book. Dr. Bresler said that chronic pain is sometimes a subconscious cry for love and tender treatment. Because people can't bring themselves to march up to someone and say directly what they want, they announce a pain (a real pain) to elicit the sympathy, the soothing touch they need. This is why one prescription that Dr. Bresler always gave his chronic-pain patients was four hugs a day. He considers these hugs so important that he even advises patients who don't have a huggee handy to approach strangers in the supermarket and hug them.

That suddenly clicked with Barbara. Hugs are even better than touches. They're more up-front, with nothing sneaky or furtive about them.

Back in the library she posted a sign on the suggestion board explaining the value of touching and hugging (lest the students consider her some kind of nut) and offered herself as hug therapist. She invited all students to drop by her desk for hug therapy whenever they had a need.

She pinned on the hug-therapist badge she'd made for herself and waited. And waited and waited. A week. Nothing. Two weeks. Still nothing. It began to look as if the hug-therapy program was also destined to trickle down the drain to oblivion.

Then one morning Barbara looked up to find a young man standing in front of her desk. He cleared his throat and swallowed. "Are you Barbara Toohey?"

"Yes."

"Well . . . er . . . ah . . . I think I could use a hug."

Barbara almost tripped over the wastebasket getting to him. They clutched each other awkwardly, blushing to the tops of their ears. But do you know what? They both felt wonderful afterward. Maybe it was partly the result of surviving a difficult ordeal, but more likely it was the hug, the human contact, the reaffirmation of identity and self-worth.

This first hug was like the first olive out of the bottle. The rest came easily. Large numbers of students and faculty members started coming into the library for their hugs. The hugging business got so brisk, especially around finals, that June and the other librarians were pressed into service as surrogate hug therapists. Several students placed themselves on a regular daily hug schedule.

Somehow the media got hold of hug therapy. (It was about the time of the Jonestown massacre and they were hungry for good news.) Hug therapy as practiced in the Los Angeles Valley College Library was on radio and TV and in the newspapers. Hugs had made a minor sweep of Southern California.

As we worked more and more with hug therapy it gradually dawned on us that this wonder drug, which is so curative for chronic-pain patients and salubrious for students, would be ideal for diabetics. In the first place, since hugging fosters a feeling of self-worth, it makes you more accepting of yourself as you are, diabetes and all. By helping you realize that you are a good person—a *huggable* person—it makes you want to take better care of that good person in order to keep that good person on the planet as long as possible. Hugging also diminishes anger—a very common emotion among diabetics—and, here we go again, it reduces stress. You can feel the tensions flow out of your body in the warmth of a hug.

We believe it would be wonderful if doctors would make it a practice to give a hug along with the diagnosis of diabetes. There is no more dismal time in your life than when you hear yourself being given that life sentence to a chronic disease, the full implications of which you can't quite grasp but nevertheless fill you with fear and uncertainty. A warm, accepting hug would be like a life preserver to hang onto at that moment. It's like the old laying on of hands that doctors used to practice before they started keeping us all at instruments' distance. The efficacy of laying on of hands might be just the placebo effect, but don't knock placebos. They have no harmful side effects and they often work. Medical science has recently discovered that placebos, like running, activate the body's endorphin system. This "morphine within" can diminish both physical and psychic pain.

As a matter of fact, all members of the diabetes-care team—nurses, dietitians, social workers—should become hug therapists on the side. Actually, hug therapists are needed everywhere in medicine. Once Barbara was visiting a friend in the hospital and forgot to remove her hug-therapist badge from the library. A dismal-looking woman who shared the elevator with her glanced at the badge and, apparently thinking Barbara was part of the hospital staff, asked, "Hug therapist? What kind of thing is that?" When Barbara explained it to her she said, "I think I'll have one." Barbara hugged her and a good measure of the gloom left the woman's face.

Hugs aren't good merely for your mental health, either. As with all the therapies we've mentioned, the mind can change the body in mysterious and wonderful ways. A recent radio report on this phenomenon amazed even us. Researchers at Ohio State University were doing a study of how diet affects atherosclerosis. As one of their experiments, they fed several groups of rabbits an extremely high-fat diet. Students were assigned to take care of these rabbits. One young woman became so fond of those in her charge that she dropped in several times a day just to pick them up and pat and squeeze them.

At the end of the experiment it was discovered that, although the rabbits in her group were eating a diet identical to that of all the other rabbits, her rabbits had only half the fatty deposits in their blood vessels.

Thinking that this was just a strange coincidence, the research team tried the experiment again. Same results. Finally, after repeating the experiment five times, they had to conclude that tender loving care did indeed do something to help prevent atherosclerotic buildup.

Hugs are as beneficial to the hugger as to the huggee. Both of us are sometimes a little shy in first encounters and find that if we announce ourselves as hug therapists and offer our services it breaks the ice better than a cocktail. After all, if you've hugged somebody it's pretty hard to be cool and distant with him or her.

There are, we must admit, a couple of small problems that present themselves in hug therapy. Some people get the wrong idea at first—especially men, who, conditioned by our culture to believe that you are never allowed to touch another person except for sex or violence, find it hard to understand a warm, human, nonsexual encounter like a hug. But we find that most of them are easily indoctrinated and often turn out to be the best huggers of all, probably because they've been deprived for so long. The other problem also concerns men. Men can hug women easily, and women can hug men. Women can also hug other women without difficulty. But, as columnist Ellen Goodman said, "There are men who would die for each other but they can't hug each other." Work on it, men. You need it and so do your friends.

When we started closing our talks to diabetes groups with hug-therapy sessions, it soon became clear that hugs and diabetics are perfect partners. We've even begun to think that, along with bike-a-thons, we should raise funds with hug-a-thons, in which you pledge a certain amount of money for each stranger the participant hugs. This would spread salubrious hugs across the nation and, besides helping finance a cure for diabetes, might even prevent diabetes complications. All the blushing that invariably goes on with hugging does tremendous things for your circulation. So get this prescription filled right away:

R_X 4 HUGS A DAY

Hug anyone in the room, anyone in the house, anyone in the library or the office or wherever you are and feel the wonder of this wonder drug.

And to send you on your way, here's one for the road.*

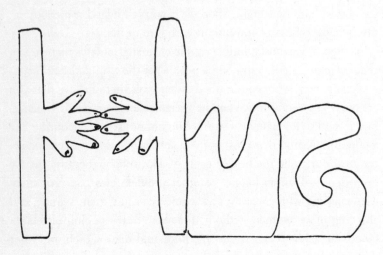

*Courtesy of Janice Kent.

CHAPTER 19

Doing unto Others

. . . .

"Be kind, for everyone you meet is fighting a great battle."

—PHILO OF ALEXANDRIA (JEWISH PHILOSOPHER)

ONE-A-DAY PLAN FOR OTHERS

A retired college professor friend told us about the time the Dalai Lama visited the campus. A few of the faculty members were invited to a private conference with him. One wise-guy professor thought he'd shake up the guest by asking what he thought would be an impossible question: "What is the purpose of life?"

The Dalai Lama answered immediately and firmly, "The purpose of life is to help others—and if you can't help them, at least don't hurt them."

This brings us to what we consider the ultimate good time and greatest source of a blithe spirit: doing something for others.

The book *At Home in Mitford* by Jan Karon is a surprise best-seller featuring a diabetic Episcopal rector, Father Tim. Every morning he utters the same prayer, "Father, make me a blessing to someone today." That's a good utterance for us all. We call it "doing-a-nice-person thing" and we make it our goal to do at least one a day.

Margaret Pickford, an eighty-three-year-old retired teacher who's had cataract surgery on both eyes, is a good example of a nice-person-thing doer. She's a volunteer who works every Monday morning in the office of Stephen Turner, M.D., an ophthalmologist in San Leandro, California. Her job is to hold patients' hands during their cataract surgery. To quote her, "Doctors and nurses may be experts in their fields, but they haven't had the surgery. That's where I have the expertise. Some people, particularly men, don't want the support at first. But they usually end up squeezing so tightly that I think my hand's coming off at the wrist." Since taking on the job, she has held the hands of about 1,400 patients. She recalls only three refusals, including a very pompous tax collector who later apologized. (We wonder why he was apologizing: For being pompous? For being a tax collector? For refusing the hand-holding? Or all of the above?)

As you gain more and more expertise in diabetes, think of the good you can do (and the pleasure you can derive) from encouraging and counseling and helping the newly diagnosed or the people who've had diabetes for a long time and are going through a patch of discouragement or experiencing harbingers of complications.

We had a diabetic friend, a talented singer, who "adopted" a little sister with diabetes. She took her on outings, invited her to plays and art exhibits, shared the pleasure of her company at lunches, and in the process subliminally showed her that diabetes won't keep you from leading an exciting, happy life and following any career your heart desires.

'Tis Blesséd to Give

Of course, giving of yourself as those above did is the greatest of gifts and the most satisfying for all concerned. But don't overlook the joy of giving of things, things you no longer need and someone else could greatly benefit from having. We have a friend who had an exercycle that was in perfect shape. She just decided to get another one, one that had a chair back so she could read and work while she pedaled. What to do with the first exercycle? She could have given it to a charitable organization and taken a deduction, but somehow that didn't do it for her. After a minimum of detective work, she found a friend who told her about a friend of *hers,* a single mother of an eight-year-old daughter, who had just gone through a rocky and rancorous divorce. The ex-husband provided zero child support. She had resigned from a very well-paying job (with long hours) and taken a less well-paying teaching assignment so her hours would coincide with her daughter's school time. She was in great need of exercise for both physical and mental health, but she couldn't afford to go to a gym and, anyway, she didn't want to leave her daughter alone. Home exercise equipment is notoriously costly. What to do? Problem solved. With the exercycle, the woman could work out at home, staying with her daughter. She even got her daughter on an early path to fitness by encouraging her to do daily pedaling on the exercycle. The woman was delighted with the gift and the giver was equally delighted, if not more so.

Give Yourself a Simpler Life

When you give away the things you no longer need (For example take diabetes equipment. How many meters do you have? How many lancing devices?), you're also giving yourself a better, simpler, uncluttered life. Enter the word "clutter" on Google or Yahoo in your computer and you'll see what an all-pervasive problem excess stuff in our lives is. As Mike Nelson says on the Clutterless Recovery website *www.clutterless.org,* "Cluttering has deep psychological and spiritual roots." And "People are important, not stuff. We have made our stuff more important in our lives than our relationships with others. When we keep that perspective, it is easier to change." And on the Free From Clutter website *www.freefromclutter.com,* we learn we can "clean physical clutter . . . as a pathway to greater productivity, effectiveness, spontaneity, creativity, vitality, and peace" in our lives—to say nothing of revving the blithness of our spirits. Bookstores are, well, *cluttered* with books on how to declutter your life. Among the most popular of these are *Stop Clutter from Stealing Your*

Life by Mike Nelson, *Lighten Up; Free Yourself from Clutter* by Michelle Passoff, *Eliminating Clutter from Your Life* by Susan Wright, and *Let Go of Clutter* by Harriet Schechter. If you get one and read it, to avoid more clutter you could then pass it on to someone else or give it to a library.

Blessing Giving

June learned about this from a *New York Times* article about poet and novelist (*The Color Purple*) Alice Walker. She has used meditation for twenty years to "conquer her inner space" and "nurture the re-creation of hope." Because of meditation she became involved with a loving-kindness meditation called "metta." This you direct toward a loved one, a benefactor, a neutral person, and a difficult person. She said that "the difficult person is always rather amusing to choose, because the moment you do so, you begin to see how much that person resembles yourself."

Should you want to send metta to someone, this is how it goes:

May you be happy.
May you be safe.
May you be peaceful.
May you have ease of well being.
(Then just to cover everything Alice adds . . .)
May you be joyful.

Above all, don't forget the metta for that difficult person, who probably needs it most of all.

ONE-A-DAY PLAN FOR YOURSELF

In *At Home in Mitford,* Father Tim, after his diabetes diagnosis, starts out going great guns on his exercise program, even going so far as to buy a forest-green running suit. But soon, under the pressure of his church duties, his resolve crumbles, and so does his exercise program. It takes a bout of nonketotic hyperglycemic coma to get him back on

track—and on insulin. Some excellent advice for all people with diabetes as well as for dedicated diabetes health-care professionals was
said to the overworked Father Tim by a fellow minister: "Sometimes
we get so worn out with being useful that we get useless."

With that thought in mind, along with the previous prescription
for "Three Hugs a Day," we offer another prescription—a pleasure
prescription. Do at least one pleasurable activity a day. Take a little
time out to do at least one thing that you enjoy, whether it's reading
part of a favorite book, calling a friend for a chat, listening to music,
practicing your putting, or just sitting in a garden watching the flowers grow.

Psychologist Tony Lysons of the University College in Swansea,
Wales, studied women in beauty parlors by attaching electrodes to
them. He discovered that when a woman gets her hair washed, cut,
and dried, not only does she look better, but her mood is measurably
improved. Her morale goes up, while her heartbeat slows and her
blood pressure goes down by 5 percent. You can extrapolate from this
how much good the beauty parlor experience will do for her diabetes
control.

CHAPTER 20

The Little Things That Count

. . . .

DAILY DELIGHTS

We all look forward to life's big pleasure events, like a wonderful vacation, an exhilarating sports activity, a moving theater experience, or whatever rows your joy boat and gives you what Barbara calls "an ecstasy attack." But while you go after the gigantic good times, make sure you get in the habit of enjoying the small daily pleasures, the little good times that keep life perking along.

The genius of the American food writer M. F. K. Fisher was her absolute insistence that life's small moments are the important ones. She once wrote a delightful essay describing nothing more than the joys of picking and cooking fresh peas on a hillside overlooking Lake Geneva. The small-daily-pleasures theory is verified by studies reported in Robert Ornstein and David Sobel's book *Healthy Pleasures:* "Many people search for happiness in the extreme highs of emotion, money, and status. And they are misled to do so. It is not those unforgettable and sought-after 'great events' or memorable successes or excesses of power that bring happiness. Instead, many small and often overlooked daily events, even trite and obvious experiences, add up in the long run."

The truth of this is illustrated in Thornton Wilder's play *Our Town*, the story of life and death in a small American town at the turn of the century. In it, Emily Gibbs, who dies in childbirth, is allowed to relive one day in her life. Her mother-in-law, who had died before her, advises her to "choose an unimportant day. It will be important enough." The excitement of returning gradually changes to sorrow and disillusionment when she sees how people—including herself—never appreciate and savor life while it's being lived, how the gift of life is not treasured and lived to the fullest. As Emily asks, "Do any human beings ever realize life while they live it . . . every, every minute?" The Stage Manager, who narrates the play, responds, "No, the saints and poets maybe, they do, some."

Thornton Wilder realized it with his belief that life is meaningful only when lived with the full awareness of the value of the present moment no matter how small or insignificant it seems at the time.

In another of his plays, *The Skin of Our Teeth*, Wilder sums it up with, "My advice to you is not to inquire why or whither, but just enjoy your ice cream while it's on your plate."

Message on a Bottle

You can find philosophy in the strangest places. We found this vintage reflection on the label of a wine bottle.

"My favorite days in life are nothing special, rather those in which I find joy in the ordinary rhythm of my existence, those in which I am simply content with my place . . . another glass of life please."

—GREG BROWN, WINEMAKER, T-VINE CELLARS, ST. HELENA, CALIFORNIA

Let's drink to that!

Changes

· · · · · · · · · · · · · · · · · · ·

"There is no pain in change; there is only pain in resistance to change."
—JUDY COLLINS, *TRUST YOUR HEART*

Now that you've traveled and adopted a pet or two and have laughed and hugged and learned the kinds of changes you can make to bring about total health and happiness, it's time to start making those changes. We're not going to tell you that it's easy to change old, bad habits to new, good ones, to switch from negative addictions to positive ones. Change—even change for the better—produces stress because it takes a lot of effort, and at first it may seem as if you're giving up all that is comfortable and pleasurable in your life.

FAIR TRADES

Trade-offs

Maybe it will help if you don't think of it as giving up things, but rather as making trade-offs. Robert Shornick, a diabetic in his fifties writing in *Diabetes Forecast,* expressed the trade-off idea in this way:

[Diabetes] made me reevaluate how I was spending my time and energy. Such a change demands trade-offs—giving up something in return for something else, not necessarily a negative exchange. Before diabetes, several drinks and a few cigarettes on an airplane after a hectic day was sheer pleasure. Another drink or two in the hotel before bed further relaxed me. Now I have a sugar-free drink on the plane and my food snack at bedtime. Not as enjoyable, but adequate. The next day my head is 10 percent clearer than it used to be. A *good trade.*

Before diabetes, my eating habits were erratic, both as to when and what I ate. Now, "when" and "what" have specific meanings for me, and my energy level has doubled. Therefore, I accomplish more. *A profitable exchange.*

Before diabetes, I weighed 158 pounds, looked a bit pudgy, and had difficulty buying suits that fit. Now I weigh 144, am trim and slim, and can find a whole selection from which to choose. *An ego-boosting trade.*

Before diabetes, my exercise pattern was sporadic, heavy on the weekends. Now I exercise daily in a programmed manner, and my body reflects a comfortable tone and hardness. Before diabetes, much time at home was devoted to necessary business activities to generate income. Now I'm working toward a better balance of work time and family time. My wife and son are the two most important ingredients in my life, so that's where I'm putting a more meaningful share of my life.

Promise Yourself a Rose Garden

There's an old saying, "Two things money can't buy: true love and home-grown tomatoes. Home-grown tomatoes are wonderful and in our vegetable garden we always had a plethora of them—enough to give away to all our friends (unlike zucchini, tomatoes are always welcome) and to cook up and freeze vast vats of tomato puree to use in sauces.

But when we went on the low-carbohydrate diet, we knew that

our wanton tomato-consumption days were over. After all, a tomato is technically a fruit and fruits are only allowed in very limited quantities—if at all. One large tomato is 8 carbohydrates and tomato puree is a titanic 25 grams of carbohydrates per cup. When you have only 30 grams of carbohydrate *all day*, tomatoes and their sauces are going to be minuscule menu items.

What to do? Well, we could go into tomato mourning and weep over their loss or we could go ahead and plant our tomato garden and succumb to the overwhelming tomato temptation and blow the diet. But luckily there was a third choice. June got the idea of plowing up the vegetable plot and planting, instead, a rose garden.

We figured we could fit twenty-four regular plants plus three climbers on the fence. We tried to get all different ones and succeeded, except for accidentally getting two Midas Touches. We didn't mind because that's one of our favorites. Luckily, June got her idea during the bare roots season, so we didn't need to have a Midas Touch ourselves to pay for them.

How has it worked out? Perfectly! Although we always enjoyed our tomatoes, we didn't have the personal involvement with them the way we do with roses. Our tomatoes were only known generically to us as "Italian tomatoes" or "cherry tomatoes" or "big red tomatoes" or "yellow tomatoes," whereas we know every rose by its proper name: Voodoo, Chris Evert, Spice Twice, Bewitched, John F. Kennedy, Kardinal, etc. And we greet each new bud with joy. Now there are always roses on the desk or table to provide a calm atmosphere during hectic days—all without carbohydrates, calories, or fat. June keeps a rose in a vase on the counter in her bathroom to give her comfort when she takes her insulin injection or checks her blood sugar. She never did that with a tomato!

The changes you must make for your diabetes—or your life—often involve giving up something. But if you put your mind and imagination to it, you'll find you can come up with something even better to replace what you lost. So promise yourself a figurative rose garden and be sure to stop and smell the metaphorical roses it produces. It's magic!

Change Busters

There will, of course, always be people who try to sabotage your efforts toward making changes. They will be happy to tell you tales such as the following true story told to June by a friend to whom she had described her new lifestyle with exercise and the low-carb diet.

This person said he had a friend who had led a freewheeling (translation: self-destructive) life up to his forties, at which time he experienced some sort of midlife crisis and decided all this had to stop. He knew he was wrecking his health with his lifestyle, which was more like a deathstyle. He did an about-face.

He gave up his six-packs and his twenty-packs. He started exercising and worked himself up to a daily five-mile run. He kept regular hours. He ate balanced meals, watching the cholesterol. (As the fellow who told the tale put it, "He gave up everything enjoyable.") He lost weight. Even the tale teller had to admit grudgingly that his friend looked great. Finally the friend even decided that his old sedentary, high-pressure job, in which he had achieved great monetary success, had to go. He quit and got a physically active outdoor job in construction work. Six months later a wayward steamroller fell on him and killed him.

The tale teller delivered the punch line with a smug, see-all-the-good-it-did-him smile on his face.

But his story did not convince us to ignore the principles of total health, and we hope it won't convince you either. Because—now hear this!—*you cannot count on having a steamroller fall on you.*

Remember the words of comedian Jimmy Durante, who stated on the occasion of his seventy-eighth birthday, "If I'da known I was gonna live dis long, I'da taken better care a myself."

Live and Learn

One of our favorite sayings of the greatest diabetologist of them all, Dr. Eliot Joslin, has always been: "Live as if you were going to die tomorrow; learn as if you were going to live forever." But now we realize that this statement is subject to misinterpretation. We assure you that "living as if you were going to die tomorrow" does *not* mean you should follow a heedless eat-drink-and-be-merry philosophy with your health. No, Dr. Joslin meant you should experience life to the fullest. To be able to do that, you have to have the best health you can. In that sense, diabetics need to live and learn as if they were going to live forever.

Live that way not *just* to keep your diabetes in control. Live that way to have the total health that will enable you to achieve happiness. And what, pray tell, is this nebulous concept of happiness? Philosophers have wrestled with that one for centuries, but no one has yet come up with what is universally accepted as the *definitive* definition. In our opinion the one that comes closest to the mark is Aldous Huxley's. As you set off on the not-always-smooth road to total health and happiness we offer it to you and wish it for you: "Love, peace, joy, and the capacity to help others."

CHAPTER 22

Farewell Sharing

JUNE'S SUCCINCT SECRETS FOR SUCCESS IN DIABETES . . . AND LIFE

Do It the Phi Bete Way

To become a good manager of diabetes, take advantage of the methods used by college students who, in their junior or senior years, are elected members of Phi Beta Kappa. This is the college honor society for the select few who have achieved the highest grades. How do these students do it? It takes dedication and good work habits as much as—if not more than—intelligence. June was Phi Betaicized in her junior year at UC Berkeley. Here she reveals to you her secrets of success so you can get straight A's in blood sugar control and become a Phi Bete in diabetes self-care.

The truth is that I had no choice. I had to develop good study habits and self-discipline out of necessity. No, more accurately, it was a matter of survival. I had a scholarship and if I didn't get high grades I would have lost it and had to drop out of college. At the same time, I had to work at least twenty hours a week for further financial support. Even so, I graduated in three and a half years instead of the usual four and I achieved all A's, except for one B in a course I took credit by examination after two weeks of study. Here are the rules I went by. I hope you will follow these rules in your diabetes care. Remember that for you, too, it's a matter of survival.

- Do what you dread most first. The thing you dread doing is often the thing you most need to do. Get it out of the way and get on with your life and other activities. You don't function well with a head full of dread. (Diabetes translation: Stop and stick your finger and take that blood sugar test even—maybe especially—when you totally don't want to. Do it now!)
- Do the hardest thing as soon as possible. (Diabetes translation: It's morning. You'd love to sleep in another hour or you'd love to have that second cup of coffee and read the paper. That would be so easy to do. It's really hard to muster your forces and get on that treadmill or exercycle or take that walk or run or go for a swim or workout in the gym. It will get even harder to do as the day goes by. This is the time to do it.)
- Do not procrastinate. (Diabetes translation: High blood sugar doesn't go away by itself. Do what you need to do to correct it *immediately.* Weight doesn't magically drop off without your doing something about it. Don't put off starting that new eating plan and exercise program until tomorrow for tomorrow never comes.)
- Work early in the day when you're fresh and rested. (Diabetes translation: Make sure you *are* fresh and rested early in the day. Don't dissipate your forces—and your future—with self-indulgent carousing that leaves a lifelong hangover.)
- Stick to the job until it's finished. (Diabetes translation: Diabetes is never finished. Never forsake your necessary personal therapies. Stick to them every day and it will be a long time before you reach the diabetes and the life finish line.)
- Discipline and a sense of priority are what it takes. (Diabetes translation: Diabetes is number 1 priority. Have the discipline to put it first even when it's inconvenient or awkward or embarrassing.)

- Don't worry about how brilliant you are; worry about how committed you are to your goal. (Diabetes translation: You don't have to be a genius to be a Phi Bete of Diabetes. As the painter William Hogarth said, "Genius is nothing but labor and diligence.")
- The Phi Bete's definition of work is "making things happen." (Diabetes translation: Make that normal A1c test happen. It may be work, but it's worthwhile and rewarding!)
- Delayed gratification is the name of the game. Work first, play later. (Diabetes translation: There will be no complications later—and lots of play along the way—if you pay attention to your self-care *now* and oh, how gratifying that will be in your future life!)

DIABETILINKS

> **DiabetiLink #1:** New Study of Happy People

The results of a recent study by Dr. Ed Diener of the University of Illinois and Dr. Martin Seligman of the University of Pennsylvania appeared in the January 2002 *Journal of Psychological Science* and were reported in the January 29, 2002, *New York Times.* Drs. Diener and Seligman took twenty-two college students who scored in the top 10 percent in several kinds of happiness tests and compared them with sixty students who came out average in the tests and twenty-two who were identified as unhappy. The "happy" ones were more social and extroverted, more agreeable and less neurotic. They spent less time alone and had strong ties with friends and family. All appeared to be satisfied with their lives, remembering more good happenings than bad ones. Strangely enough, the study shot down some long-established what-increases-happiness theories. The happy group didn't exercise more than those lower on the scale nor did they sleep more or attend church more often. Incidentally, even those in the happiest group were not constantly blissed-out. They experienced some down moments, but that's not all bad because, as Dr. Deiner pointed out, unpleasant emotions not only signal that something is wrong, but motivate people to make necessary changes.

Dr. Seligman makes an important point. His theory is that there are probably different kinds of happiness. One deals with "the giggles and pleasures and joys of life" and the other with what Aristotle called "eudaemonia," which can be translated as "good spirit" and is the result of "an active life governed by reason."

Our theory is that if you have "an active life governed by reason," especially relating to your diabetes self-care, then you're more likely to get your fair measure of the "giggles and pleasures and joys."

(Return to p. 5.)

➤**DiabetiLink #2:** For Veteran Blood-Sugar Testers

New and improved meters are constantly coming on the market. You can often even get one free with a trade-in. There is one warning, though. The older meters give whole blood readings but some, in fact many, of the newer meters give plasma readings. Meter companies are making this change because then the readings on their meters will line up better with the labs that give you your A1c test results because the labs give plasma readings. When you switch meters you may find your blood sugars appear to be higher. Remain calm. *Diabetes Self Management* gave these comparison guidelines to show how your new goals would be compared to the old ones.

	WHOLE BLOOD GOAL	PLASMA GOAL
Blood sugar before meals	80-120 mg/dl	90-130 mg/dl
Blood sugar at bedtime	100-140 mg/dl	110-150 mg/dl

(Return to p. 10. If you want to skip all the blood-sugar testing information go to page 24, but really you shouldn't skip this information. You may learn about something important such as the new GlucoWatch and you may be encouraged to be more regular in your testing if perhaps over the years you've grown casual and complacent.

➤**DiabetiLink #3 for Type 1's:** Improvements in Insulin and Insulin Injecting, Rationale for Multiple Shots, New Developments in Control

THE MORE THE MERRIER

Multiple shots—or at the very least two shots a day—are the cornerstones of good diabetes therapy. A personal aside. June currently takes four shots of insulin a day: One of Humalog, the fastest-acting of the fast-acting insulins, before each meal and one Lantus at bedtime. She also takes an additional small amount of Humalog when she runs a "surprise" high blood sugar. She gives the multiple shots much of the credit for the fact that after thirty-six years of diabetes she has no complications.

We want to give a word of praise for the two newest members of the insulin family: Humalog and Lantus. Humalog has been with us a few years now and it was a most welcome addition to the insulin smorgasbord. As nurse Virginia Valentine puts it, "It works like we always wished regular would work." That is to say, it works so quickly that you can take it when you sit down at the table and in only fifteen minutes it starts lowering your blood sugar. About the time you've finished the meal—an hour to an hour and a half—it's at its peak of effectiveness. Then in two to four hours when you no longer need it, it goes away and doesn't bother you anymore. Now there's another FDA member of the rapid-acting insulin family: Novolog (aspart). It works with the same speed as Humalog and, although to this date there have been no head-to-head tests with Humalog, it's safe to assume that the two insulins will be comparable in their action and duration.

Lantus (glargine), which just came on the scene in the spring of 2001, is an equally important breakthrough. Instead of taking two shots of NPH (morning and night), you only need to take one of Lantus at bedtime, since it covers your basic bodily functions (basal) needs for twenty-four hours. (Anything that eliminates a shot from your daily life is a welcome friend.) Better still, unlike NPH, it doesn't have peaks of activity that can cause unexpected low blood sugars at inappropriate moments—is there ever an appropriate moment? Another plus is you don't have to roll the vial to mix it before each shot the way you do NPH.

It is said that some people find it stings a little on injection, but June doesn't find it so. Maybe because she's so happy with its other features that she just doesn't notice.

Based on June's experience and that of other diabetics as well as our reading in diabetes literature, we long believed that you can't have good control with one shot of NPH a day. But we saw so many diabetics who were on that therapy and who stoutly maintained that they were doing just fine, thank you very much, on one shot and who claimed that their doctors said that was all they needed, that we bit our tongues and said nothing. But at an ADA conference in Wichita, Kansas, we heard one of the nation's most respected diabetologists, Richard Guthrie, speak and he stated flat out that *good control is not possible on one shot of NPH a day.* This is because, as he explained it, while the life of NPH insulin may be twenty-four hours, its therapeutic life (the period during which it controls blood sugar) is only about thirteen hours. With one shot of NPH, therefore, you have eleven hours during which your blood sugar may not be controlled.

This reminded us of the representative of a Danish insulin company, who used to squirm at lectures by a well-known diabetologist who was, himself, diabetic. The doctor would point sternly at the rep and say "It's all your company's fault that there are so many diabetics with complications like blindness and kidney failure and amputation." The company's founder had been the one who, years ago, first developed NPH. At that time everyone hailed NPH as a great breakthrough because it meant that rather than taking one shot of regular before each meal, diabetics could take one shot of NPH in the morning and forget about it for the rest of the day. Since blood-sugar monitoring was not possible in those days, the one-shot-of-insulin people didn't realize they were running around with high blood sugar a good part (make that a bad part) of the time. The lecturing doctor maintained that many of these people could have avoided the complications they later developed had they been taking insulin the old-fashioned way with a shot of regular before each meal.

But it's not just the dreaded complications of diabetes that can be avoided with tighter control (frequent blood-sugar tests and insulin injections three or four times a day). A Harvard study of 1,400 type 1 diabetics reported at the American Diabetes Association sixty-first Scientific Session (June 2001) showed that diabetic patients who follow this tighter regimen develop less atherosclerosis (artery-clogging plaque) than those who test and inject insulin only once or twice a day and these cardiovascular benefits continue over the long term. As Dr. David Nathan, co-chairman of the study, said, "When you treat patients early, you slow the momentum of atherosclerosis. It's as though you've made them six years younger. You take away that much of their diabetic history." The diabetic fountain of youth apparently flows with insulin!

Now there are many effective insulin therapies using combinations of regular or Humalog and NPH or Ultralente or Lantus. Your doctor can work out the best kind of therapy for you based on how your body works and the kind of life you lead.

In his talk, Dr. Guthrie provided the dismal statistic that up to 80 percent of insulin-taking diabetics are still on one shot of NPH a day. Don't you be one of them.

NO PAIN, NO STRAIN

To make you ready and able, and most important, willing, to take a more effective number of insulin injections, many less painful and more convenient ways of injecting insulin have been developed:

1. Devices that shoot the needle into you quickly and virtually painlessly. These include:

   Autoject and Autoject 2 (these also deliver the insulin when they insert the needle) Owen Mumford 1-800-727-6500, www.owenmumford.com
   BD Automatic Injector Becton-Dickinson 1-888-232-2737, www.BD.com/diabetes

Instaject Medicool 1-800-433-2469, www.medicool.com
Inject-Ease Palco 1-800-346-4488, www.palcolabs.com

2. Penlike devices for injecting small amounts of insulin by click-
   ing or twisting. With these you can inject the number of units
   you want without having to fill a syringe ahead of time. This
   is extremely convenient when you're injecting before meals
   away from home. These include:

   Autopen Owen Mumford 1-800-727-6500,
      www.owenmumford.com
   BD Pen Becton-Dickinson 1-888-232-2737,
      www.BD.com/diabetes
   Disetronic Pen Disetronic Medical Systems 1-800-280-7801,
      www.disetronic-usa.com
   Humalog Pens (Note: these are available in Humalog and
      several combinations of Humalog and longer-lasting
      insulins.) Eli Lilly 1-800-545-5979, www.lillydiabetes.com
   NovoPen 1.5, Novolin Prefilled, and NovoPen 3
      NovoNordisk 1-800-727-6500, www.novo-nordisk.com

3. Jet Injectors. These are a boon for the truly needle-phobic
   since there is no needle involved, just the small, focused
   stream of insulin. Using a jet injector can make for better control because the insulin goes right into action since it doesn't
   "pool" at the injection site as it often does with needle injection. These are more expensive than needles and you might
   have a struggle with your insurance plan (what else is new?!) to
   get them to cover one. Thorough instruction is particularly
   important with these. The currently available jets are:

   Advanta Jet, Advanta Jet ES, and **Gentle Jet** (appropriate for
      children and very thin adults) Activa Products
      1-800-991-4464, www.advantajet.com
   Injex 30 Equidyne Systems 1-877-474-6539, www.equidyne.com

Medi-Jector Medi-Ject 1-800-328-3074, www.mediject.com
Vitajet 3 Bioject 1-800-848-2538, www.bioject.com

4. Pumps. This—with a little help from the wearer—mimics the action of the pancreas, delivering you a preprogrammed continuous rate of basal (covering basic bodily functions) insulin and then at mealtime you press a button to release a bolus (larger amount) of insulin to cover the meal. A pump is more expensive and more complicated to use than injecting the old-fashioned way and it requires as many if not more blood-sugar tests. But it gives a huge amount of freedom. You can bolus and join the dinner party when everyone else is ready to eat. You can change time zones with ease. You can engage in sports activities by adjusting for the greater amount of exercise. Most are waterproof for watersports activities.

There are many diabetics—especially younger ones—who seldom if ever could achieve anything near good control with conventional injections but were put right on track with a pump. For this reason some of the skinflintiest insurance plans and HMOs are willing (after the usual and customary Great Struggle and mountains of paperwork) to subsidize the purchase of a pump and its on-going supplies.

June's insulin therapy as previously described is commonly called "the poor-person's pump" because it mimics the action of the pump as it mimics the action of the pancreas.

Just as with meters, there are constantly new developments on the pump scene. You will probably want to select the one recommended by your diabetes health-care team since they will be the ones showing you the ropes and helping you with the programming and solving any problems that may develop. The currently available pumps are:

Animas R-1000 and **AnimasR-1000A** Animas Corporation
    1-977-YES-PUMP, www.animascorp.com
D-TRON, H-TRONplus Disetronic Medical Systems
    1-800-280-7801, www.disetronic-usa.com

MiniMed 508 MiniMed Technologies 1-800-933-3322, www.minimed.com

If you're considering going onto a pump, you should read one (or more!) of the following:

* *The Insulin Pump Therapy Book: Insights from the Experts,* Introduction by Jay S. Skyker, M.D.
* *Teens Pumping It Up* by Elizabeth Boland, MSN, APRN, PNP, CDE
* *Optimal Pumping: A Guide to Good Health With Diabetes* by Linda Fredrickson, M.A., R.N., CDE, Richard R. Rubin, Ph.D., CDE, and Stefan Rubin

The above books can be ordered from Medtronic/MiniMed 800-843–6687 or *www.minimed.com.*

* *Pumping Insulin* by John Walsh, PA, CDE and Ruth Roberts, M.S.

This can be ordered from the Diabetes Mall 800-988–4772, Fax 619-497–0900, or *www.diabetesnet.com.*

THE NOSE HAS IT

Because we want to alert you to possible good things to come, we want to mention Exubera, an insulin inhaler not yet FDA approved but currently being tested. With this, you inhale a dry powder form of insulin, which is absorbed into the body through an aerosol made by Inhale Therapeutics. Early trials showed that it was as effective as injected insulin. But there have been possible side effects in the trials, including one case of pulmonary fibrosis (scarring of the lungs) and four of pulmonary effusion (a buildup of fluid in the lungs). The *New York Times* Health & Fitness section reported that "Doctors involved in the studies said they did not think that the drug caused the pulmonary fibrosis or three of the cases of pulmonary effusion. The fourth case is still under investigation."

Patients involved in the study "overwhelmingly preferred using the inhaled to the injections" according to Dr. Alan Moses who is one of the investigators and the chief medical officer at Boston's Joslin Diabetes Center.

To keep up with the developments you can search the Web under the name "Exubera." And watch the news for other unusual non-needle insulin delivery systems. Before long there will be others. (Return to p. 19.)

> **DiabetiLink #4 for Type 2's:** Taking Your Diabetes Seriously, Testing More than You Want to, New Developments in Control, Scared Straight

Dr. Richard Guthrie had some wise words of caution for type 2 (non-insulin–taking) diabetics. Type 2's have a tendency to think of themselves as having "mild" or "borderline" diabetes . . . (This misinformation is sometimes spread by well-meaning health-care professionals who don't want to upset their patients with a full-blown "you've got diabetes" diagnosis.) It's only human to think it's not as serious as type 1, because you don't have to take insulin. Push that reassuring thought from your mind. Type 2 diabetics have a different kind of diabetes, but they, in their own way, are just as diabetic as type 1 and should take their diabetes as seriously and take just as good care of themselves as their insulin-taking brethren and sistren. This includes taking blood-sugar tests. Dr. Guthrie points out that type 2's' blood sugars can fluctuate during the course of the day just as much as type 1s' and unless they take frequent blood sugars (fasting and before and after meals) and provide their doctors with the data on their fluctuations, the doctor cannot prescribe the correct dosages of oral hypoglycemic pills and/or make the dietary adjustments necessary for the good control that keeps complications away. Yes, sad to say, type 2 diabetics *can* develop complications just like type 1's if they don't keep their blood sugars in the normal range. The vascular damage can begin when the blood sugars are consistently over 150 milligrams per deciliter and, as Dr. Guthrie points out, this is just as true for both type 1 and type 2 diabetics.

WHAT'S THE DIFFERENCE?

Although type 1's and type 2's both have similarities in their need for control they do have marked differences that make some experts theorize that in a sense they are two different diseases. Type 1's are insulin *deficient.* They make no insulin—or not enough of it—and therefore have to inject insulin to survive. Type 2's, on the other hand, make plenty of insulin, sometimes too much. Their problem is that they're insulin *resistant*—the insulin has a hard time getting into the cells. Often type 2's can control their diabetes with diet and exercise, but if, despite their best efforts, their blood sugars remain high, then oral hypoglycemics (pills that lower blood sugar) are brought into play. Currently there are fifteen different kinds of these and they approach the high–blood-sugar problem in different ways. Two of the most frequently used hypoglycemics are the sulfonylureas, which incite your pancreas to send out more insulin and Metformin (Glucophage), which reduces the production of glucose in the liver. You and your doctor can work with them singularly and in combination until your blood sugar is normalized.

What if these pills don't work—or gradually stop working? Sometimes they can be helped along with a single shot of NPH or the new Lantus insulin at bedtime to see if that will give you the much-desired normal fasting blood sugar (first blood sugar in the morning before breakfast), which usually sets the pattern for the day.

SCARED STRAIGHT

Once at a diabetes conference we heard a doctor tell about a cow study in which the cows had to line up three times a day, extend their tongues, and take an oral hypoglycemic agent. A person in the audience interrupted him, "Excuse me, doctor," he said, "but how in the world were you able to get those cows to line up and accept those pills three times a day?"

"It was easy," responded the doctor, "I told them if they didn't do it, I'd put them on insulin." Of course this was a bit of diabetes humor, but it is fraught with the truth that the universal diabetic dread is having to go on to insulin. What can happen is if blood sugars remain consistently and constantly high over the years, is that the pancreas keeps pumping out more and more insulin trying to bring the blood sugars down. Finally, the poor old pancreas gets worn out from all this effort and just gives up, a victim of what the noted endocrinologist Lois Jovanovic graphically calls "pancreatic poop-out." When this happens you are no longer a type 2: you have moved into the type 1 (insulin-taking) camp.

We're not telling you this to frighten you. We just want to convince you of the importance of taking your diabetes seriously and following your therapy scrupulously. Sometimes it takes the incentive of the fear of the needle to convince a person—just as it did the cows—that it's well worth the effort of conscientiously following an exercise program and a diet plan, and whatever else is prescribed to keep your blood sugar normal. If that is the incentive it takes, take it. (Return to p. 19.)

> **DiabetiLink #5:** The Healthy Eating Pyramid

Walter Willett, M.D., chairman of the Department of Nutrition at the Harvard School of Public Health and a professor at Harvard Medical School, is the author of *Eat, Drink, and Be Healthy: The Harvard Medical School Guide to Healthy Eating*. In this book he criticizes the Department of Agriculture's pyramid as being "built on shaky scientific ground," "wishy-washy"—and "flat-out wrong." At worst, he says that the information it offers contributes to obesity, poor health, and unnecessary early deaths.

He objects to its being more weighted toward dairy products, red meat, and breads, a distortion, he believes, probably caused because it was produced under the auspices of the Department of Agriculture (USDA), the agency that is responsible for promoting agribusiness, rather than under the agencies responsible for promoting and monitoring health.

Some of his primary differences with the USDA pyramid include:

* The USDA pyramid tells you to use fats sparingly but ignores the fact that two kinds of fat, monounsaturates and polyunsaturates,

found in olive oil and other vegetable oils, whole grains, and other plant products are good for your heart.

• The USDA lumps all complex carbohydrates together to form the base of the pyramid rather than recognizing that the *type* of carbohydrate is important. Whole grains in breads and pastas should be specified. White bread, potatoes, pasta, and white rice may be complex carbohydrates, but the digestive system turns them into glucose and sends this sugar to the bloodstream almost as fast as taking pure glucose. In the Healthy Eating Pyramid, potatoes have been moved out of the vegetable category and into the "use sparingly" category because of their dramatic effect on levels of blood sugar and insulin.

• Dr. Willett objects to the USDA pyramid giving equal protein billing to red meat, poultry, fish, eggs, beans, and nuts. He believes red meat a poor choice because it contains saturated fat and cholesterol. It may also give you too much iron whether you need it or not.

• The USDA pyramid has too heavy an emphasis on dairy products—two or three servings per day. As a prime source of calcium they are supposedly there to fight the "calcium emergency" that threatens Americans' bones. But in truth, Americans get more calcium in their diets than people in all other nations except Holland and the Scandinavian countries. There is little evidence that getting high amounts of calcium prevents broken bones in old age. And now there are studies indicating that consuming great quantities of dairy products may increase chances of ovarian cancer in women and prostate cancer in men.

• The Healthy Eating Pyramid allows moderate alcohol consumption (one drink per day for women, two for men) to reduce the chances of heart attacks, heart disease, and strokes. It also recommends taking a multivitamin "insurance policy" and has an important base-line recommendation of daily exercise and weight control.

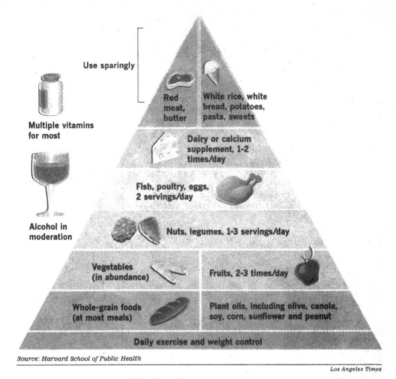

The Healthy Eating Pyramid
(Return to page 40)

➤ DiabetiLink #6: Dr. Bernstein's Chart of Food Conversion to Glucose

Approximate Timing for Digestion, Conversion to Glucose, and Appearance as Increased BG

FOOD TYPE AND CONVERSION PROCESS	BG RISE BEGINS	LAST TRACE OF GLUCOSE APPEARS IN BLOOD
Glucose. No digestion required. Moves directly through stomach and intestinal walls into bloodstream.	2 minutes	½ hour
Fructose (fruit sugar). No digestion required. Moves into bloodstream through intestinal walls. Converted by liver to triosephosphates, which also are intermediate products of glucose metabolism. These will convert to glucose if not covered by additional insulin.	25 minutes	1½ hours

	Approximate Timing for Digestion, Conversion to Glucose, and Appearance as Increased BG	
FOOD TYPE AND CONVERSION PROCESS	BG RISE BEGINS	LAST TRACE OF GLUCOSE APPEARS IN BLOOD
Sugar alcohols (used as artificial sweeteners, also found in fruits and vegetables). Converted in a manner similar to fructose.	25 minutes	1½ hours
Sucrose (table sugar). Digestion breaks the glucose molecule away from the fructose molecule. The two separate molecules then proceed as above with the original glucose portion appearing as BG first.	5 minutes	1½ hours
Starch and other polysaccharides. Salivary (and pancreatic) amylase breaks down much of it to maltose, which is further degraded to glucose in the small intestine.	10 minutes	1½ hours
Protein. Denatured by acids in stomach, then broken down into amino acids by digestive enzymes in small intestine. Amino acids enter bloodstream and those not used for tissue building are converted to glucose by the liver.	1½ hours (If we ignore the Phase I glucagon effect that can be offset by relatively low blood levels of insulin)	4 hours
Fat. Is not converted to glucose. There does exist a Phase I glucagon effect if consumed in large amounts. This can be offset by relatively low blood levels of insulin.		

Reprinted by permission from *Diabetes: The GlucoGraf Method for Normalizing Blood Sugar*, by Richard K. Bernstein (Los Angeles, Jeremy P Tarcher, Inc., 1983).

(Return to p. 54.)

▶ DiabetiLink #7: A Pinch of Salt

Once when we chirped merrily about how we had just about totally given up salt, instead of offering congratulations, Dr. Bernstein issued a warning about what happened to his aunt when she became a salt abstainer. We contacted him again for more details for this book. This was his response:

> Since I told you about my aunt, who had postural hypotension secondary to dehydration, I've observed many, many instances of

this condition amongst my patients and even my mother and mother-in-law. I see this most commonly in elderly individuals [Surely he can't be referring to eternally youthful *us!*] who avoid the consumption of fluids and salt. The problem usually occurs in hot weather when they are losing fluid through perspiration and are not replacing it adequately. They become dehydrated. Since their blood volume is diminished for lack of water, they are unable to deliver enough blood to the brain. This problem is especially common in people with diabetes because of sympathetic neu-ropathy that prevents arteries in their legs from closing down when they stand. This automatic or, more appropriately, auto-nomic reflex prevents blood from pooling in the legs and depriv-ing the brain. When such dehydrated individuals stand up, they get light-headed and feel like they are going to pass out. The body holds onto water better if salt is not restricted.

Dr. Bernstein refers you to pages 273 and 274 of his book, *Dr. Bern-stein's Diabetes Solution,* for a related discussion. (Return to p. 77.)

➤ **DiabetiLink #8:** Extremism in the Reduction of Fat Is No Virtue
The American Heart Association has long advocated that we keep our dietary fat to under 30 percent. Some heart specialists (notably Dr. Dean Ornish) have advised heart patients to restrict fat to only 10 or 15 percent. But a new controversy has erupted with a report saying that cutting fat back this much may not ease heart risk at all. (*Circu-lation, Journal of the American Heart Association* September 1998). In fact, according to the American Heart Association's May 1998 Advi-sory Statement, "At this time, no health benefits and possible harmful effects can be predicted from adherence to very low-fat diets in certain subgroups." Subgroups include persons with insulin-dependent dia-betes and those with hyperinsulinemia (in other words, type 2's).

This same warning holds true for persons with eating disorders and the elderly. The main concern is that this diet may elevate triglyceride levels and at the same time reduce the levels of HDLs ("good" cholesterol). Yet another hazard is that, though you may lose weight on an extremely low-fat diet, you could be at risk for malnutrition or, as health professionals call it, "nutrient inadequacy."

(Return to p. 82.)

➤**DiabetiLink #9:** No Joy in Soyville

A well-meaning e-mail pen pal in Hawaii sent us an article by Helen Altonn from the November 19, 1999, *Honolulu Star Bulletin.* It had the following lead in, "Too much tofu induces 'brain aging' study shows. A Hawaii research team says high consumption of the soy product by a group of men lowered mental abilities."

The article went on to explain that Dr. Lon White of the Pacific Health Research Institute revealed that a Hawaii study showed a significant statistical relationship between two or more servings of tofu a week and "accelerated brain aging" and even an association with Alzheimer's disease.

Not only were the above deleterious results of eating tofu revealed, but the claims of the benefits of soy made by the food-supplements industry were pretty much shot down. Particularly cited were their claims that "isoflavones, plant chemicals found in high concentrations in soybeans, offer 'natural' cures for breast cancer, osteoporosis, prostate cancer, heart disease, menopausal 'hot flashes' and other chronic conditions."

Dr. White stated that "the majority of scientists said the data they were talking about for the beneficial effects on health is very weak and doesn't really support health claims for soy foods."

But the Fickle Finger of Food Facts immediately geared up for another fast swivel. A letter-to-the-editor in the *Register* suggested that the tofu used in the tests may have been processed with chemicals and *they* were responsible for the negative results, not the tofu, itself.

And to give tofu a small nudge back into the tent of approval, in the February 2000 issue of *Diabetes Forecast,* there was an article in the Healthy Living section called "Soy Power." As it said on the cover, it's "One Health Food You Shouldn't Ignore." The article explained that "while the actual mechanisms and amount of soy that are beneficial to health are being researched, some of the findings seem very promising." The examples given were: keeping bones strong (reducing osteoporosis), lowering the bad (LDL) cholesterol, relieving hot flashes, and lowering cancer risk.

We continue to have tofu as part of our diet. (Return to p. 89.)

➤ DiabetiLink #10: Oh Say Should You C?

After an era of almost universal acceptance, they're starting to knock vitamin C. Researchers in Britain have discovered that a supplement of 500 milligrams a day could damage people's genes. You know how we've all been advised to take C for cold prevention and antioxidant benefits? The study by pathologists at the University of Leicester found in their six-week study of thirty healthy men and women that a daily 500-milligram supplement had *pro*-oxidant as well as anti-oxidant effects on the genetic material DNA. Antioxidants block molecular damage caused by molecules known as "free radicals" and protect against heart disease, cancer, cataracts and other chronic health problems. Pro-oxidant, on the other hand, cause genetic damage by promoting the generation of free radicals from iron in the body. It would seem that the benevolent vitamin C has an evil twin.

American doctors studying vitamin C also warn against large doses, pointing out that the vitamin C naturally present in foods are the best way to get the vitamin. The U.S. recommended daily intake of vitamin C for healthy adults is only 60 milligrams, easily obtained in foods. The British team concluded that normal healthy individuals would not need to take supplements at all.

For years we've been taking one gram (1,000 milligrams) of C daily. Those naughty free radicals must be jumping for joy as they run around damaging our DNA. And yet Linus Pauling, that great advocate of C who took 12,000 milligrams a day, lived to the age of 93.

(Return to p. 94.)

➤ DiabetiLink #11: The Water Tide May Be Turning

Benedict Carey, health writer for the *Los Angeles Times* in his convincing anti-mainstream article "Hard to Swallow" asks the question "Should healthy adults really be stalking the water cooler to protect themselves from creeping dehydration?" He then delivers the answer "No!" in thunder from well-qualified experts in the field.

"The notion that there is widespread dehydration has no basis in medical fact," states Dr. Robert Alpern, dean of the medical school at the University of Texas Southwestern Medical Center in Dallas.

Carey points out that most nutritionists don't know where such an idea came from. He quotes Barbara Rolls, a nutrition researcher at Pennsylvania State University, as saying, "I can't even tell you that, and I've written a book on water."

Jurgen Schnermann, a kidney physiologist at the National Institutes of Health, believes that "an average-size adult sitting in a temperate climate needs no more than one liter of fluid." That's only four 8-ounce glasses—exactly what Barbara came up with on her own.

Based on a study by researchers at the Center for Human Nutrition in Omaha, Carey also sinks the idea that drinks with caffeine don't count in your daily requisite liquid tally. The study's lead author, nutritionist Ann Grandjean, says flatly of the idea that caffeine is dehydrating, "It is not." Drinks containing alcohol do produce a loss of fluids but it takes more than one drink "to cause noticeable dehydration."

Other revelations include the fact that drinking copious quantities of water doesn't curb your appetite or improve your skin; you can get a great deal of your daily water requirements in your food (soups, fruits, and vegetables, and thirst actually *will* usually tell you when you need to drink more.

You really should read all of Carey's watershed article. You'll find it on the Internet if you noodle around on either Google or Yahoo under the name "Benedict Carey." You might make a copy of it and press it into the free hand of friends who are clutching a water bottle with the other.

Humorous aside: When Barbara called the *Los Angeles Times* to find out if Benedict Carey was male or female, she was put straight through to him (as it turned out). Barbara took the opportunity to compliment him on his excellent, well-researched article. She then asked him how he came up with the idea for it. He was partially inspired by his parents, he said, "who are in their seventies and in very good shape, and I never saw them drink anything except coffee and Scotch."

(Return to p. III.)

➤**DiabetiLink #12:** Chart of Calorie Expenditures

	GROSS ENERGY COST (CALORIES PER HOUR)
REST AND LIGHT ACTIVITY	**50–200**
Lying down or sleeping	80
Sitting	100
Driving an automobile	120
Standing	140
Domestic work	180
MODERATE ACTIVITY	**200–350**
Bicycling (5½ mph)	210
Walking (2½ mph)	210
Gardening	220
Canoeing (2½ mph)	230
Golf	250
Lawn mowing (power mower)	250
Bowling	270
Lawn mowing (hand mower)	270
Fencing	300
Rowboating (2½ mph)	300
Swimming (¼ mph)	300
Walking (3¾ mph)	300
Badminton	350
Horseback riding (trotting)	350
Square dancing	350
Volleyball	350
Roller skating	350

VIGOROUS ACTIVITY	OVER 350
Table tennis	360
Ditch digging (hand shovel)	400
Ice skating (10 mph)	400
Wood chopping or sawing	400
Tennis	420
Waterskiing	480
Hill climbing (100 ft per hr)	490
Skiing (10 mph)	600
Squash and handball	600
Cycling (13 mph)	660
Scull rowing (race)	840
Running (10 mph)	900

Reprinted from *The Diabetic's Sports and Exercise Book,* by June Biermann and Barbara Toohey (Philadelphia, J.B. Lippincott, 1977).

(Return to p. 138.)

➤**DiabetiLink #13:** Flying with Diabetes Supplies

New aviation safety guidelines require people with diabetes who carry diabetes supplies to take the following rules into account:

- Passengers may carry insulin and syringes or other insulin delivery systems (e.g., a pen or pump) only if they can produce an insulin vial or package with a pre-printed pharmacy label that clearly identifies the medication. Pen users will need to keep and carry the box in which the pen comes, and syringe and pump users will need to keep the boxes from their insulin vials.
- For people who test their blood sugar but do not use insulin, lancets may be carried onto aircraft as long as the individual lancets are capped (unused) and are brought with a blood-glucose meter with the manufacturer's name embossed on the meter.
- Glucagon must be in the original packaging with the pre-printed pharmacy label clearly visible.

- Prescriptions for medications *will not* be accepted in lieu of original packaging with pre-printed pharmacy labels, due to the possibility of forgery.

In the event that you encounter problems boarding a flight, you should contact the FAA grounds security commissioner at the airport for assistance. You should not pack diabetes supplies in checked baggage, because the cargo hold temperatures can vary greatly and because you may need the supplies during the flight. (Return to p. 204.)

> **DiabetiLink #14:** The Best of Mary

ANIMAL MAGNETISM

A True Pet Tale

My psychologist friend Dr. Richard Rubin told me a true story in which an animal taught a family with an eight-year-old diabetic daughter an important lesson. Their pet dog had a litter of puppies, one of which was born with a club foot. The father was talking to his daughter about it. "I think we'll have to put that puppy to sleep." (Don't you just love that euphemism?) The girl was very upset and protested that she didn't know why they'd have to do such a thing.

The father explained, "You see he has that bad foot and he can never have a happy life with a problem like that." The little girl, now in tears, said, "You think he can't have a happy life just because there's something wrong with his foot? There's something wrong with me, too. I have diabetes but I know that I can still have a happy life."

Of course, the father saw the light and relented, and the puppy and the girl are living happily ever after despite their "flaws."

This story has particular poignancy for me because I have a club foot, too—my right rear paw. Actually no one ever notices my foot. They're too busy looking at my ears, which, since I am a Scottish Fold, are folded over and close to my head. I wish I had a can of tuna for every time I've heard someone say, "What's wrong with your cat's ears?"

The truth is, none of us is perfect, and a good thing, too. A man named Leonard Cohen wrote a song called "Anthem" in which he says, "There's a crack in everything. That's how the light gets in."

The Dead Cat in the Temple Syndrome

Now you may think this is a rather depressing topic, but stay with me and you'll see that I'm giving you another way to get rid of your worries and enjoy life to the fullest. It has to do with what psychologists call "catastrophizing." This just means looking at a situation and making the worst possible interpretation of it. This story was told to me by June and Barbara, and they swear it's true. I believe them because we've always had an honest and forthright relationship and I know they wouldn't lie to me.

This event took place when they were visiting Hong Kong a few years ago. One day they went to the Man-Mo Temple, the oldest temple in the city. It is the temple of the god of literature and they thought Man-Mo might give them some help with their writing. (I, of course, need no such divine intervention for my talents.) At any rate, as they wandered through the temple they came upon a woman in one of the chapel areas. She was kneeling before the altar and praying. Next to her on a satin pillow was a ginger-colored cat, who was lying absolutely still.

The woman was not praying silently. In fact she was shrieking hysterically. As June and Barbara stood there in the shadows feeling sorry for the woman, her prayers got wilder and wilder. They didn't want to intrude on her agony, so they moved on, but each in her own mind had the same interpretation of why the woman was in such apparent distress. They both thought the immobile cat had just died and she had brought it to the temple to pray for its feline soul or even to try to get the gods to bring her beloved pet back to life.

After wandering through a few more small chapels, they felt irresistibly drawn back to the drama of the woman and her dead cat. The woman was gone, but the cat was still there. She raised her head to look at the commiserating pair, got onto her feet, yawned, stretched, and ambled off on some cat errand or other. They figured that she must be the temple cat who slept whenever—and wherever—she pleased, including on satin altar pillows.

After leaving the temple they discussed the situation and decided that the woman probably wasn't all that disturbed. As they had noticed in restaurants and on the street, Cantonese with its up and down intonations, has a tendency to sound as if people are excited or upset when they're just carrying on a normal conversation or even, presumably, praying.

At any rate, now when they look at a situation and start giving it the most negative interpretation possible, they stop and say, "It's just a dead cat in the temple." Then they laugh and go about their business. I hope you can use this technique to laugh away some of your needless worries, too. And I also hope you never see a real dead cat!

Tough Love for the Diabetic Man, Woman, Child, or Cat in Your Life

When I went to my vet, Dr. Garner, for my annual checkup and shots, he told me about one of his patients. It was a cat with out-of-control diabetes. This fellow weighed around nineteen pounds and looked like one of those blown-up balloons in the Macy's Thanksgiving Day parade. (I, myself, weigh less than nine and believe me I'm not just fur and bones.) Dr. Garner put the cat on insulin and told the cat's person that she would have to feed the cat carefully measured food only two times a day. The woman looked dubious because she always kept a bowl of food available so the cat could eat any time he felt like it, but she said she'd try.

The next time she came in with the cat he was as fat as ever and his blood sugar was as high as ever. Dr. Garner couldn't understand why nothing had changed so he asked the woman if she had been limiting her cat's food. "No," she said, "because he screams bloody murder if I don't give him more food when he wants it." It made her feel too cruel, so she always gave in and fed him.

"There must be something else you can do." She said accusingly to Dr. Garner. He said he didn't know of anything to control diabetes except limiting food and balancing the insulin, but if she wanted another opinion . . . He gave her the name of another vet—a very expensive vet!—who specialized in endocrinology. She went off happily.

A couple of months and $1,200 later she was back again. The specialist had told her exactly the same thing so she was finally doing it and the cat's screams were gradually diminishing and so was his weight. His blood sugar was also getting under control. She learned that Dr. Garner's therapy was right—and his prices reasonable.

The lesson here is that sometimes you have to be tough to be truly loving. Keep that in mind whenever you want to give in and indulge the diabetic in your life—even if that diabetic is you, yourself.

Incidentally, Dr. Garner was recently in the hospital for some surgery, and a not-too-adroit nurse had trouble getting a needle into his vein. She jabbed and jabbed and jabbed. Finally Dr. Garner lost patience with her and said, "If I did that to my patients, they'd bite me." Maybe that's an idea. If you don't like the kind of treatment you're getting, start biting. I, personally find it very effective.

Pets Make You Healthy

There are two means of refuge from the miseries of life: music and cats.

—ALBERT SCHWEITZER

Albert Schweitzer was right! When you're feeling bad, there's nothing like having your cat around to comfort you. Someone recently sent June a cat greeting card by *Pet Tales* that said, "Cats know exactly how we feel—they don't give a damn, but they know." That, of course, is just a joke. *We know and we care—a lot!*

But we—and our other animal colleagues—do more than care. Just the other day when I happened to be reading the publication *The New Scientist,* I came across the following item: "Evidence continues to mount that pet owners live longer, healthier lives than those who are petless. A British study found that within months after acquiring a cat or dog, new pet owners suffered less from headaches, backaches, and flu. An Australian study found that pet owners tend to have lower cholesterol levels than non-pet owners with comparable life styles. Convincing, isn't it?

But what if you don't have a pet and don't even want one? Well, I suggest that you get one and you'll soon find you love it. Radio Psychotherapist Dr. Toni Grant explains, "You love the thing you take care of. If you have the ugliest, dumbest damn dog around and you feed it and give it water and baths and take it for walks, you'll soon find yourself loving it." Get a pet and you'll see that Dr. Toni is right.

Note: I sincerely apologize for the profanity in this column. I assure you I don't talk like that, myself. I wasn't brought up that way. But as a conscientious journalist I feel I must quote others accurately.

Half a Pet Is Better than None

But if you can't bring yourself to get a whole pet, how about half of one. I don't mean you should saw the poor creature in half, but rather that you share custody with someone else. I read about this on radio consumer advocate Clark Howard's website. He quoted a *New York Post* article that told about "the latest trend in the city whereby two people or families share a dog. One owner has the dog in the day, the other gets it at night or some other arrangement." That sounds wonderful to me. It's particularly nice for older people who might not have the energy to walk the dog as much as it needs. (We cats can handle our own walking, thank you very much, not to mention our own bath taking.) The article did warn that there would have to be an agreement about food costs and vet bills and such, but surely that could be worked out in a fair way. And if you want to do a double good deed, you could adopt a retired racing greyhound. They make wonderful pets and get along beautifully with people and other animals, including cats and birds and hamsters. For information call Greyhound Pets of America, 1-800-366-1472.

With love from your true friend, Mary,

(Return to p. 223.)

AN ECLECTIC COOKBOOK FOR PEOPLE WITH DIABETES AND THEIR FAMILIES AND FRIENDS

PART 5

The word *eclectic* has many meanings: "selecting or choosing from various sources," "using what are considered the best elements," and "chosen for its fanciful appropriateness." All the meanings apply here.

We've selected and modified these recipes from various sources: favorite cookbooks, favorite national cuisines, favorite restaurants, favorite friends, and favorite successful experiments we've made in the kitchen. Admittedly, a few of these recipes may contain a tad more fat than you—or we—normally put in dishes. But these are special treats that you won't be having every day or every week or every month. Even so, don't hesitate to cut back further on fat to stay within your recommended diet. The dishes will still be good.

In the recipes, we use what we consider the best elements—the best ingredients and the best methods of preparation and serving.

We like to think of them all as *fanciful.* The one thing we think food should never be is boring. That's why we've included only dishes that please and tickle our food fancies. We hope they'll do the same for yours.

BASICALLY NOT BASIC

This is by no means a basic cookbook—a complete compendium like the *Joy of Cooking*—or what we consider the diabetic equivalents of that honored tome, *The Art of Cooking for the Diabetic;* or even the four volumes of *The American Diabetes Association/American Dietetic Association Family Cookbooks.*

No, this eclectic collection won't bring you from not knowing how to boil an egg to preparing a state dinner for the prime minister of France. And yet in another sense it *is* basic. We've tried to explain the recipes in such a way that even a very inexperienced cook could handle them. In some cases where the recipes verge on the time-consuming or complex, we've given a simpler alternative that sacrifices very little in the ultimate enjoyment.

AROUND A DIFFERENT WORLD

In the very first edition of our very first diabetes book, *The Peripatetic Diabetic,* we included an "Around the World Cookbook," including our favorite dishes from different cuisines. We still like international dishes, but the culinary world we explore now is a kinder, gentler-on-your body place with lower fat and sodium and higher fiber. Also, back in those days, when it came to eating out, very expensive French restaurants were about the only places you could find a variety of vegetables prepared in interesting ways. Now our tastes lean toward relatively inexpensive Italian restaurants, and our recipes, with a great emphasis on things Italian, reflect that change of taste. It has been said that when you're in love, the whole world's Italian. It holds equally true that when you're in love with cooking, if the whole world is not Italian, at least a very large part of it is.

PLAY WITH YOUR FOOD

When we encourage you to play with your food, we're not advocating that you draw happy faces in your mashed potatoes or flip spoonfuls of peas at your dining companions. No, we mean that when it comes to cooking, you should be relaxed and happy and make variations on dishes depending on what's in season and what you have in the house.

We ourselves used to be so rigid that when we were making a recipe—especially for the first time—we'd run all over town trying to find exactly the called-for ingredients. Not only did this result in a state of exhaustion and irritation that took away the pleasure of the cooking and eating, but often the dish didn't turn out as well as it would have if we'd played with the recipe using, for example, ingredients that were in season and readily available.

Being flexible with your ingredients is also a thrift measure. What we ordinarily do is take whatever protein (generally the most expensive part of the meal) is on sale and build dinner around that.

Ultimately your greatest fun comes when you become confident and experienced enough in the kitchen to decide you don't want to go out—either to a restaurant or to shop for ingredients—and just make dinner out of what you can find around the house. When you manage to turn out something you've never had before and it's something wonderful, your dining pleasure multiplies exponentially.

COME INTO OUR KITCHEN

Now, after this preamble, we invite you to try some of these favorite recipes of ours. We hope you will read them with excitement and anticipation, prepare them—for yourself and others—with love and enthusiasm, and dine upon them with pleasure and joy. For each recipe, we provide you with the nutritional information and diabetes exchanges for one serving of the basic recipe. These were calculated for us by Lambert, DeVito, Bauersfeld and Associates, Registered Dieticians. Optional variations that we suggest or that you make will differ slightly.

However, one of our goals with this little cookbook for diabetics is to free you from feeling you have to use *only* cookbooks for diabetics. We hope that as you work your way through these recipes, you'll start to become familiar enough with ingredients that you will be able to estimate fairly closely what the exchanges are in any and all recipes you may want to try. After all, that's what the exchanges are— fairly close estimations (just as the blood-sugar tests you make are only fairly close estimations). To tell the truth, after twenty-five years of following the so-called diabetic diet, we hardly ever use cookbooks specifically designed for diabetics anymore. The one exception we make is when it comes to desserts, which often take quite a bit of delicate balancing of ingredients to deliver the correct texture and sweet taste without excessive calories.

In most cases we've given you the information on how to find special ingredients that we suggest, but if you have trouble locating any of these, write to us at 5623 Matilija Avenue, Van Nuys, CA 91401, and we'll do our best to track them down for you.

· Breakfast ·

Most of us prefer something familiar and comforting for the first meal of the day, and that's why we stick to more standard American fare at breakfast. There are few things more familiar and comforting than muffins. We're including two of our favorite recipes here. These are good not just for breakfast, but for a midmorning snack, too.

BREAKFAST BRAN MUFFINS

MAKES 8 MUFFINS

These are our basic breakfast muffins, which June bakes almost every week. Often we even take a batch with us on trips, for breakfast in the hotel room. They are chock-*full* of fiber, and you know how hard it is to get your fiber when traveling—or even at home, for that matter. Miller's bran (not bran cereal) is available in boxes in some supermarkets and in all health-food stores.

1 cup whole wheat flour
3 teaspoons baking powder
½ teaspoon salt (optional)
1 cup bran
2 tablespoons vegetable oil

2 tablespoons Fruit Sweet*
   or molasses
1 egg
1 cup nonfat milk
Raisins (optional)

Heat the oven to 425 degrees. Sift together flour, baking powder, and salt (optional). Add bran and stir thoroughly. In a separate, smaller bowl mix together vegetable oil, Fruit Sweet (available from Wax Orchards; phone 1-800-972-2323) or molasses, the egg, and milk. Add this to the dry ingredients and mix only enough to moisten. Fill Pam-sprayed muffin tins, or tins lined with paper baking cups (we spray these), two-thirds full. Bake for 15 minutes, or until done. As a variation you can add the raisins, either to the whole batch or to half of it.

8 SERVINGS   EXCHANGES PER SERVING: 1 starch; 1 fat   CALORIES: 142
PROTEIN: 6 gm   CARBOHYDRATE: 23 gm   FAT: 5 gm   FIBER: 4 gm
CHOLESTEROL: 27 mg   SODIUM: 268 mg

L.A. FITNESS MUFFINS

MAKES ABOUT 16 MUFFINS

We call these L.A. Fitness Muffins because we keep them in the freezer and have one before going to a workout at our gym (L.A. Fitness Center). But they're really good any time, and since they have some fruit built in, you can enjoy them au naturel. You have your choice of fruit, but do your taste buds a favor and use fresh, not canned, fruit.

*Wax Orchards, 1-800-634-6132, 22744 Wax Orchards Road SW, Vashon Island, WA 98070
www.waxorchards.com

*1 cup blueberries (or halved
   cherries, diced peaches,
   or raspberries)
1¾ cups all purpose flour,
   sifted
½ teaspoon salt
2 teaspoons double-acting
   baking powder
3 tablespoons granular fructose
   (available in health-food stores)*

*1 egg
1 egg white
2 tablespoons avocado or other
   vegetable oil
¾ cup nonfat milk
1 teaspoon grated orange or
   lemon rind*

Prepare the fruit first by lightly flouring it. Preheat the oven to 425 degrees. Sift together the flour, salt, and baking powder. Add the granular fructose and mix thoroughly. In a separate bowl beat the egg and egg white; add the avocado oil, milk, and the grated orange or lemon rind. Add the wets to the dries and blend partially before dropping in the fruit. The entire stirring process should not take more than 20 seconds (there may be some lumps). Fill Pam-sprayed tins two-thirds full; bake 20 to 25 minutes.

16 SERVINGS   EXCHANGES PER SERVING: 1 starch   CALORIES: 80
PROTEIN: 2.5 gm   CARBOHYDRATE: 12 gm   FAT: 2 gm   FIBER: 0.6 gm
CHOLESTEROL: 13.5 mg   SODIUM: 122 mg

You can make wonderful muffins the super-easy way using a prepared blue corn muffin mix available from Natural Choices, Inc. (505-242-3494). They also make a dandy blue corn pancake and waffle mix.

Usually for breakfast, though, we just have cereal of some kind—in warm weather usually a cold cereal such as Fiber I or Breakfast O's (Barbara's Bakery). In cold weather it's oatmeal or oat-bran cereal. We have two favorite oatmeals: McCann's Irish Oatmeal (the non-quick-cooking variety), which we first discovered when we had breakfast at Rumpelmayers before taking our morning walks in Central Park. (We like to live dangerously!) When time is short you can make a delicious quick-cooking oatmeal that's available from Christine and Rob's (41103 Stayton Scio Road SE, Stayton, OR 97383–9406; phone 503-769-2993), www.christineandrobs.com. They also have a wonderful old-fashioned baking-powder biscuit mix that makes a lovely Sunday breakfast.

DR. RON BROWN'S ROYAL CANADIAN OAT BRAN

SERVES I

Oat bran is a little out of style compared with what it was a few years back, but it shouldn't be out of your diet. Just ask Dr. Anderson (see page 40). Not only does oat bran vacuum up cholesterol, but it really sticks to your ribs and every other bone in your body. You feel full for hours, which makes it great for people who are on a weight-losing program.

Dr. Ron Brown, our first employee, is a dietitian as well as a doctor and a magnificent cook. This recipe shows how he took something prosaic and turned it into something really wonderful.

⅓ cup oat bran
½ cup nonfat milk
½ cup water
Dash salt
½ small or ¼ medium green
   apple

1 packet Equal
2 dashes cinnamon
1 tablespoon roughly chopped
   peanuts
1 tablespoon raisins
1 teaspoon sugar-free syrup

Combine the oat bran, nonfat milk, water, and salt in a small saucepan. Heat to boiling over medium-high heat. Reduce heat and simmer for 3 minutes. While it simmers, put the following into your cereal bowl: the apple, Equal, cinnamon, peanuts, raisins, and sugar-free syrup like Maple Grove Farms' Cozy Cottage, St. Johnsbury, VT 05819, www.maple-grove.com. We add cooked oat bran and stir to combine.

I SERVING   EXCHANGES PER SERVING: I starch; ½ milk; 2 fruit
CALORIES: 245   PROTEIN: 12 gm   CARBOHYDRATE: 47 gm   FAT: 7 gm
FIBER: 8 gm   CHOLESTEROL: 2.2 mg   SODIUM: 204 mg

· Herbaceous Lunches ·

In California we're fortunate that salad greens are easy to come by year round and not hard to grow yourself. People make a lot of fun of Californians and their radicchio and arugula and endive and mache, but in truth these greens do enliven a salad and bring it out of the ordinary. Arugula is the easiest of all to grow yourself, since it's officially classified as a weed, but it's very expensive to buy in the market and even more so in a restaurant. Another easy grower that brightens up the taste of the other greens is mint: chop up a few leaves (not enough to overwhelm) for your mixed green salad and taste the difference. Of course, any other herbs you may have in your garden or pots are welcome: basil, chives, oregano, marjoram, thyme, tarragon. All you need for these salads is a light dressing of oil and vinegar; we like to add a little Dijon mustard to further perk things up.

There are two other slightly more complex salads we particularly enjoy.

A TOTALLY UNAUTHENTIC CAESAR SALAD

SERVES 4

Despite arguments to the contrary, Caesar salad was invented in Tijuana, Mexico. We know this for a fact because Barbara was there with her father and had one when she was in junior high. Mexican in origin as it may be, the Caesar salad has been rattling around the United States—especially California—for so long and has gained so much popularity that we've adopted—and adapted—it as our own. Everyone has his or her favorite way of fixing it and claims it to be the most authentic. There is, for example, a raging controversy concerning the inclusion of anchovies. We've heard that Caesar's daughter claims her father would never consider putting anchovies in his. One thing every "authentic" Caesar salad has is a raw or coddled-for-one-minute egg. Ours doesn't. We've taken seriously the warnings about salmonella in uncooked or even undercooked eggs. So here is our recipe, unauthentic as all get-out, but we think you'll like it. We do.

1 large head romaine lettuce
2 or 3 anchovies or a 3-inch strip
* of anchovy paste*
½ teaspoon cracked black
* peppercorns*
⅓ cup extra-virgin olive oil
¼ cup grated Parmesan cheese
1½ tablespoons red-wine
* vinegar*
1 tablespoon freshly squeezed
* lemon juice*

1 to 1½ tablespoons pressed or
* minced garlic*
1 teaspoon dry mustard
½ teaspoon celery salt (optional)
3 dashes Tabasco sauce
⅓ teaspoon Worcestershire sauce

GARNISH:
Niçoise-style olives
Freshly grated Parmesan cheese
Grated egg white

Wash and dry the lettuce. (We like to use one of those plastic salad spinners, but Barbara's father used to meticulously dry each leaf with a dish towel.) Put it in the refrigerator until ready to toss.

Into a blender or food processor with a metal blade (we prefer the former) put the anchovies or anchovy paste (you can leave out the anchovies if you really hate them, but they blend with the other ingredients and don't make the dressing taste like anchovies), peppercorns (you can crack these with a rolling pin or use a peppermill if you have one that has a setting loose enough to crack rather than grind), olive oil, Parmesan cheese, vinegar, lemon juice, garlic, dry mustard, celery salt, Tabasco sauce, and Worcestershire sauce. Blend thoroughly.

You can either tear the leaves of romaine into pieces and toss, or leave the leaves whole and spoon the sauce over the leaves. Either way, go easy on the dressing: you don't want a puddle of Caesar soup in the bottom of the salad bowl or plate. We like to garnish the salad with a few small black Niçoise-style olives and, if you can afford the fat, some more grated Parmesan or, preferably, some Parmesan shaved from a piece. We sometimes give a nod to the traditional egg by grating some egg white into the bowl before tossing, or grating it on top of the whole-leaf salad.

We usually forgo the traditional croutons since they have extra carbohydrate and fat. June prefers to just have a crusty piece of French bread with it. One of the advantages of not having a raw or coddled egg in the dressing is that if you don't use all the dressing you can keep it in the refrigerator and use it later on without fear.

If you're absolutely forbidden any cheese at all, you can leave it out. When you do, the dressing will be strikingly similar to the dressing used on the next recipe.

ONE TABLESPOON DRESSING   EXCHANGES PER SERVING: 1½ fat
CALORIES: 74   PROTEIN: 1.5 gm   CARBOHYDRATE: 1 gm   FAT: 7 gm
FIBER: 3 gm   CHOLESTEROL: 2.5 mg   SODIUM: 173 mg

COBB SALAD

SERVES 4

Cobb salad was supposedly born when there was a lack of the wherewithal for a standard chef's salad. It is basically a chopped salad of whatever greens, vegetables, and protein you happen to have on hand. We've made some wonderful unauthentic Cobb salads in just this way—and like them just as well as the more standard variety. But remember that the variations on this theme can be infinite, and if you don't have or can't find all the ingredients—especially all those different greens—just use what you *do* have and *can* find.

¼ head iceberg lettuce
½ bunch watercress
1 small bunch curly endive
    or chicory
¼ head romaine lettuce
1 tablespoon minced chives
1 medium tomato, peeled,
seeded, and diced
1 cooked chicken breast
1½ hard-boiled eggs, diced
1 or 2 strips bacon (optional)
¼ cup Roquefort, Gorgonzola,
    or blue cheese (optional)

DRESSING:
¼ cup water
¼ cup red-wine vinegar
¼ teaspoon sugar equivalent of
    granulated fructose or artificial
    sweetener
1½ teaspoons freshly squeezed
    lemon juice
½ teaspoon salt (optional)
½ teaspoon black pepper, preferably
    freshly ground, fairly coarsely
¼ teaspoon English or Dijon mustard
½ large or 1 small clove garlic, minced
¼ cup extra-virgin olive oil
¾ cup vegetable oil

Finely chop and place in a large bowl the lettuce, watercress, endive or chicory (we've sometimes used regular endive and/or fennel), romaine lettuce, chives (or, if you don't have them, green-onion tops). Place the tomato, chicken, and egg in the bowl on top of the greens.

The authentic recipe also calls for a slightly more necessary (as far as flavor is concerned) evil: bacon. Rather than using the recommended 3 strips, we use 2 (if Barbara's making it) or 1 (if June is). We wrap the strips (or strip) in paper towels and zap until crisp and dry in the microwave and crumble on top of the other salad ingredients. Another fat bearer is also supposed to be crumbled onto the salad: ¼ cup Roquefort, Gorgonzola, or blue cheese. Let your conscience—and your cholesterol—be your guide here. Chill the ingredients until serving time.

This recipe yields way more dressing than you'll need, but you might as well make a lot of it and keep it in the refrigerator to use later. Place all the ingredients in a jar (the better to shake in later). Chill the dressing. When you're ready to serve the salad, shake the shucks out of the dressing and put just enough on the salad to lightly coat the ingredients. Put in just a little at first. You can always add more, but you can't take it out. Toss the salad and serve.

4 SERVINGS USING 1 TABLESPOON DRESSING PER SERVING
EXCHANGES PER SERVING: ½ vegetable; 1½ medium-fat meat; 3 fat
CALORIES: 206   PROTEIN: 12 gm   CARBOHYDRATE: 3 gm   FAT: 15 gm
FIBER: 1 gm   CHOLESTEROL: 107 mg   SODIUM: 325 mg

Incidentally, if you want to make this a main course and need more protein, just throw in another diced cooked chicken breast.

· Dinner Dishes from Around the World ·

<u>UNITED STATES</u>

COMFORT ME WITH MEAT LOAF

SERVES 4

In the chaotic modern world, many of us are turning to comfort foods, things that make us feel warm and cozy and taken care of the way we were when we were children (if we were lucky!). One of the most popular comfort foods is meat loaf. It's even appearing on the menus of some of Los Angeles's most trendy restaurants such as 72 Market Street and Engine Company Number 28. Like most Americans, we love meat loaf. We love it hot, we love it even more cold; we love it as a main course and we love it in sandwiches. We've tried dozens of recipes over the years, and although all are delicious—it's hard to make a bad meat loaf—we've settled on *this* one because it's exceptionally easy, different, and tasty.

2 eggs, beaten
½ cup finely chopped onion
2 tablespoons drained bottled
    horseradish
4 tablespoons rolled oats (not
    the instant variety)

1½ pounds ground chuck
2 tablespoons ketchup
Salt and freshly ground pepper
    (optional)

Stir all the ingredients together in a bowl. (A healthy variation is to use half ground turkey and half lean chuck. When we do this we add 1 teaspoon of beef-stock-base crystals or a ground-up beef-bouillon cube to give it more flavor.) Form into two 3-by-5-inch loaves, place in a shallow baking pan, and bake at 400 degrees for half an hour. Note: if you prefer, rather than putting the ketchup into the mixture, you can put it on top just before baking. It's good either way.

4 SERVINGS   EXCHANGES PER SERVING: 1½ medium-fat meat
CALORIES: 110   PROTEIN: 8 gm   CARBOHYDRATE: 2 gm   FAT: 7 gm
FIBER: 0.26 gm   CHOLESTEROL: 54 mg   SODIUM: 52 mg

MASHED POTATOES WITH GREEN ONIONS

SERVES 4

For total comfort the only thing to serve with meat loaf is mashed potatoes. In fact, mashed potatoes are the ultimate comfort dish. This healthy version, flavor-heightened with scallions, is so fast and easy that you now have no excuse to *ever* again use instant mashed potatoes, which are a whopping 80 on the Glycemic Index

2 russet potatoes   *1 tablespoon melted butter*
⅔ cup nonfat milk   *¼ cup chopped green onions*

Microwave the potatoes in the usual way (wash, prick with fork, wrap with a paper towel, cook between 5 and 10 minutes until they yield to a gentle squeeze; turn once halfway through the cooking period). Remove from the oven and let rest (still wrapped) for 5 minutes.

Next, in a 1-quart microwave bowl, put milk, butter, and green onions (you can also use chives) plus a little salt and pepper. Microwave uncovered at high for 2 minutes. Peel the potatoes and put them through a ricer or the medium disk of a food mill and add to the milk-and-green-onion mixture. Stir well, adding a little more milk if you prefer a softer consistency.

4 SERVINGS   EXCHANGES PER SERVING: 2 starch; ½ fat   CALORIES: 150
PROTEIN: 4 gm   CARBOHYDRATE: 27 gm   FAT: 3 gm   FIBER: 2 gm
CHOLESTEROL: 8 mg   SODIUM: 58 mg

CRAB (AND JUST ABOUT ANY FISH) CAKES

SERVES 6

If June ever played that game about what you would order for your last meal on earth, there's no doubt what she would select: crab cakes. She's never been known to pass one up on a menu. Not that she hasn't had some losers—greasy and with more bread crumbs than crab. But she's had some winners, too. Among those that live in the annals of her crab-cake memory are those from the Fog City Diner in San Francisco, Obrycki's in Baltimore, and (surprise!) the Hyatt Dulles just outside Washington, D.C. June likes crab cakes so much that we frequently make them at home and sometimes make them when we don't have any crab. We've made this recipe with fresh crab, canned crab, and frozen crab. We've made it with half crab and half canned tuna when we didn't have enough crab on hand. We've made it with all canned tuna when that was all there was. We've made it with fresh salmon—especially when it's on sale (poaching it first in water with a slice of lemon, a few peppercorns, a clove, and some parsley). And—maybe the best way of all—we've made it with alder-smoked salmon from Oregon, available from many mail-order catalogs. We've even made it with whatever leftover fish we've brought home from restaurants in doggie bags. So here it is. Make it any way you like. Just make it!

1 large egg, beaten
1 tablespoon low-fat mayonnaise
4 drops Tabasco sauce
1 tablespoon lemon juice
1 teaspoon Worcestershire sauce
⅛ teaspoon ground cloves
½ teaspoon paprika
¼ teaspoon dry mustard
2 tablespoons green onions, minced
Salt and freshly ground pepper to taste
1 pound crab meat
3 tablespoons dry bread crumbs or cracker crumbs
2 tablespoons oil

HORSERADISH SAUCE:
3 tablespoons low-fat mayonnaise
1 teaspoon drained bottled horseradish
1 tablespoon minced fresh parsley leaves

SHERRY CAYENNE MAYONNAISE:
3 tablespoons low-fat mayonnaise
1 teaspoon dry sherry
Cayenne pepper to taste

HERBAL SPICE MAYONNAISE:
3 tablespoons low-fat mayonnaise
1 teaspoon (or more to taste) Arizona Herbal Spice Dip Mix

In a bowl combine egg, mayonnaise, Tabasco sauce, lemon juice, Worcestershire sauce, cloves, paprika, dry mustard, green onions, salt and freshly ground pepper to taste. Lightly but thoroughly stir in crabmeat (or whatever fish or combination of fish you will). Add dry bread crumbs or cracker crumbs. (If the mixture seems excessively moist, add just a few more crumbs.) Form into 6 patties. Keep them as light as possible; don't pack them down into dense disks. Let them rest, uncovered, on foil or wax paper for around 15 minutes.

Heat oil in a nonstick pan and sauté over medium heat until golden brown on one side; turn and do the same thing on the other side.

Serve with lemon wedges or one of the following sauces. For Horseradish Sauce mix together the mayonnaise, horseradish, and parsley. For Sherry Cayenne Mayonnaise mix together the mayonnaise, dry sherry, and cayenne pepper. Or use the Herbal Spice Mayonnaise, which is particularly good on salmon cakes because it has dill in it. Mix mayonnaise and 1 teaspoon (or more to taste) of Arizona Herbal Spice Dip Mix (available from Arizona Champagne Sauces and Mustards, phone 1-800-342-9336). Make this at least half an hour prior to serving so the seasonings (which are dehydrated) can blend into the sauce.

Note: if you make fish cakes frequently, you can vary the taste by making the Maryland style (substitute 1 teaspoon Old Bay Seasoning for the other spices) or Mexican style (add 1 teaspoon minced canned green chiles—not jalapeño; they're too hot for this) or curried (add ½ teaspoon curry powder).

6 SERVINGS   EXCHANGES PER SERVING: 2 lean meat; 1 fat   CALORIES: 126
PROTEIN: 13 gm   CARBOHYDRATE: 3 gm   FAT: 6 gm   FIBER: 0.2 gm
CHOLESTEROL: 87 mg   SODIUM: 317 mg

THE PACIFIC RIM

We feel particularly blessed to live in a Pacific Rim state. We're a Western gateway to the East as well as a gateway from the East through which pass exciting cuisines. We can try these in restaurants or, if we're lucky, go through the gateway and try them in the countries themselves and then reproduce them in our own kitchens.

INDIA

JAQUA CHICKEN TANDOORI

SERVES 8

Here's yet another Indian chicken dish; if any country has taken chicken out of the prosaic, India has. This version was given to us years ago by one of our colleagues, Los Angeles Valley College home-economics professor Ida Jaqua. It never disappoints us or our guests. It's also extremely low in fat since the skin is removed from the chicken before cooking and you grill or broil it without oil.

2 chickens, quartered,	*1 teaspoon coriander*
broilers of approximately	*1 teaspoon saffron threads*
2½ pounds each	*¼ teaspoon cayenne pepper*
1 medium onion, chopped	*¼ teaspoon cinnamon*
1 pint plain nonfat yogurt	*¼ teaspoon cloves*
½ cup fresh lime juice	*¼ teaspoon nutmeg*
1 teaspoon salt	
2 teaspoons powdered ginger	GARNISH:
1 teaspoon turmeric	*Slices of onion and lime*
1 teaspoon cumin	

First you skin the 2 broilers, which you have split into quarters. Make three slashes on each piece so that the marinade can penetrate. Arrange the chicken in a single layer in a large baking pan (not aluminum).

The marinade is made in a food processor. First chop the onion and put it aside. Then put into the processor the yogurt, lime juice, salt, ginger, and spices. Blend this with an on-and-off motion until smooth. Add the chopped onion and mix well.

Pour the marinade over the chicken, turning to coat on all sides. Cover the pan with foil or plastic wrap and place in the refrigerator for 12 to 24 hours. (We have cheated on this time recommendation and the chicken still had plenty of flavor.)

The final step is to barbecue the chicken on your grill—unless, of course, you own one of those marvelous tandoori ovens that you see in the better Indian restaurants. We have the next-best thing on our patio, a Kamado-Hibachi Pot—an earthenware oven made by an ancient Japanese process.

Remove the chicken from the refrigerator 30 minutes before cooking. Place pieces on an oiled barbecue grill or under your oven broiler rack and cook 12 to 15 minutes on each side. To test for doneness, pierce the thickest part with a knife point. Escaping juices should be yellow, with no trace of pink.

Arrange the chicken pieces on a large platter in an attractive pattern. Garnish with onion and lime.

8 SERVINGS   EXCHANGES PER SERVING: 3 lean meat; ¼ skim milk
CALORIES: 154   PROTEIN: 27 gm   CARBOHYDRATE: 3 gm   FAT: 4 gm
FIBER: 0 gm   CHOLESTEROL: 115 mg   SODIUM: 138 mg

You can serve your tandoori chicken with basmati rice, which has a nice perfumy flavor. But if that's not available in your area, Dr. Brown's recipe is a good and exotic alternative.

DR. BROWN'S WILD AND BROWN RICE PILAF

SERVES 4

½ cup raw wild rice
½ cup raw short-grain
 brown rice
2½ cups chicken stock
2 tablespoons minced parsley

1 cup coarsely chopped
 mushrooms
Freshly ground pepper
4 tablespoons lightly toasted
 almond slivers

Combine in a medium-size saucepan: wild rice, brown rice, stock, parsley, mushrooms, and pepper to taste. Cover, bring to a boil, and simmer for 1 hour. During the last 5 minutes, stir in the almond slivers. Makes approximately 2 cups.

4 SERVINGS   EXCHANGES PER SERVING: 1 starch; 1 fat   CALORIES: 149
PROTEIN: 5 gm   CARBOHYDRATE: 24 gm   FAT: 4 gm   FIBER: 3 gm
CHOLESTEROL: 0 mg   SODIUM: 501 mg

To round out your Indian feast, here's a vegetable recipe we picked up in Sri Lanka. It's named not after the detective in the raincoat, but after the capital city.

SPINACH COLOMBO

SERVES 2

1 tablespoon vegetable oil	*¾ teaspoon powdered coriander*
1 medium onion, minced	*1 large bunch chopped spinach*
1½ teaspoons cumin	*2 chopped tomatoes*

In a large skillet or wok, heat the oil and slowly cook the onion until soft. Add the cumin and coriander. Stir until mixed with the onion. Increase the heat and add the spinach a little at a time, stirring constantly. When all the spinach has been added, add the tomatoes (slice across the equator and squeeze out the juice and seeds before chopping). Cook uncovered, stirring occasionally, for 3 minutes.

2 SERVINGS EXCHANGES PER SERVING: 1½ fat: 2 vegetable
CALORIES: 115   PROTEIN: 3 gm   CARBOHYDRATE: 11 gm   FAT: 7 gm
FIBER: 4 gm   CHOLESTEROL: 0 mg   SODIUM: 57 mg

CHINA

DIM SUM

We'll start our cooking adventures in China—the way they sometimes start the eating adventures in midmorning—with dim sum (also sometimes spelled *deem sum* because it's pronounced that way). Dim sum seems to gain a lot of meanings in the translation. We've read it as "heart's delight," "little jewels that tug at the heart," "heart warmers," and "little heart."

We first encountered dim sum in Japan, when we were at lunch in a Chinese restaurant. Women were pushing steam trays and carts around the room, and people were selecting dishes from them and eating happily. We couldn't order any because we didn't know what was in them (we spoke neither Japanese nor Chinese). Later research revealed that dim sum were varied items such as deep-fried egg rolls, yeast buns filled with vegetables or meat, various ingredients in thin dough, plus some things too unusual to describe.

To be honest, June doesn't like going to dim sum restaurants because she has trouble calculating her meal, especially in cases when she has no idea what she's eating (it could be a disguised chicken foot). Barbara, of course, loves dim sum restaurants. Now we usually compromise and create them at home. It's not hard to do, but it is a bit time-consuming.

What we suggest is to make a whole lot at once and freeze the ones you don't use; then later, when you take them out, you have an effortless treat. Also, rather than eating a whole pile of dim sum for a meal, we use a couple of them for appetizers and then follow up with a stir-fry dish such as the Crab in Black-Bean Sauce we tell about later. Sometimes the wonton coverings and the vegetables in the meal provide enough carbohydrate so you don't need to have a separate serving of rice, or else just a very small one (4 wonton wrappers are 1 Starch/Bread Exchange).

MAINLY SHRIMP SIU MAI

MAKES 24 SIU MAI

This is sometimes spelled *shu mai* (again because that's how it's pronounced). *Siu mai* are little pouches of good stuff—sometimes pork, sometimes shrimp, sometimes a combination of those. Here's one of our favorites.

Happily, with the internationalization of America you can probably find wonton skins in your market. They're a real drag to make because you have to make them so thin, and thin is important in wonton skins—specially for diabetics.

1 pound raw shrimp
6 dried Chinese mushrooms
6 water chestnuts (canned)

1 tablespoon low sodium soy sauce
1 tablespoon dry sherry

3 tablespoons bamboo shoots 1 teaspoon sesame oil
  (canned) 1 egg white, beaten
3 green onions 24 wonton wrappers
8 ounces lean pork

For the *siu mai* filling, clean the shrimp, removing the shell and cutting down the outside rounded part to remove the black vein. (A special shrimp knife helps a lot here.) If your shrimp are tiny, keep out 24 of them; if they're medium, keep out 12; if they're pretty big, keep out 8. If they're *huge,* keep out 6. Chop the rest of the shrimp.

Soak the Chinese mushrooms in hot water for half an hour. Remove and throw away the stems and chop the caps into small pieces. Also chop the water chestnuts, bamboo shoots, and green onions. Mince the pork. Combine all the chopped and minced ingredients in a bowl. Add the soy sauce, sherry, sesame oil, and beaten egg white. Mix well. Now the fun begins.

Take a wonton wrapper and place either in the palm of your hand or in the circle made by joining your thumb and index finger. Place a heaping teaspoon of the filling in the center of the wonton skin, and gather the sides up around the filling in pleats so that it looks like a little money bag. There will be an open space at the top into which you will insert a tiny shrimp (or ½, ⅓, or ¼ of a larger one). Put the filled wrappers into a pan or bowl and cover with a damp towel. Proceed until you've made 24 *siu mai.* Put the ones you're using for that meal into a steamer, which has been lightly oiled. Cover and steam for 20 to 30 minutes. Serve either hot or cold, with dipping sauces (see on page 306).

4 SIU MAI EXCHANGES PER SERVING: 2 medium-fat meat; 1 starch; ½ vegetable CALORIES: 276 PROTEIN: 31 gm CARBOHYDRATE: 23 gm FAT: 5 gm FIBER: 2 gm CHOLESTEROL: 164 mg SODIUM: 212 mg

POTSTICKERS

MAKES 24 POTSTICKERS

Another variety of *little hearts* we like to make are potstickers.

*¾ pound beef or pork, finely
  minced or ground*
1 pound Chinese celery cabbage
*1½ teaspoons low sodium
  soy sauce*
*½ teaspoon sugar equivalent of
  fructose or artificial sweetener*

1 teaspoon vegetable oil
1 egg white
24 wonton skins

TO COOK:
1 tablespoon vegetable oil
½ cup water

Mince the Chinese celery cabbage (or savoy cabbage or, in desperation, regular cabbage), sprinkle with salt, wrap in a cloth or dish towel, and squeeze out as much of the liquid as you can. Combine in a bowl the finely minced beef or pork, cabbage, soy sauce, fructose or artificial sweetener, and vegetable oil (if you like the taste of sesame oil, use that).

Lightly beat the egg white. Use a Joyce Chen plastic "Dumplings Plus" press or the one made by the Frugal Gourmet or a generic equivalent. Place the wonton skin over the dumpling press, put a teaspoon of filling in the middle, brush the outer edges with egg white (to make them stick), close the dumpling maker firmly, and remove the potsticker, putting it on a board or plate covered with a damp towel. If you don't have a dumpling maker you can just put the filling into the middle of the wonton skin, brush the edges with egg white, and press around the edges with a fork. Continue making potstickers until you've used up all the filling. Freeze the potstickers you aren't going to use at once.

Put 1 tablespoon of vegetable oil in an 8- or 9-inch *nonstick* frying pan that has a lid. We emphasize nonstick because the first time we made these, we used a regular frying pan and learned the true meaning of the term *potsticker.* Heat the oil over a medium flame and arrange the potstickers in a circle; they can touch one another. Add

½ cup water to the pan, cover, and cook over medium heat until the water has evaporated. This should take around 6 or 7 minutes. Turn the heat down to low and continue cooking with the lid still on for another 2 or 3 minutes, or until the dumplings are golden brown (but not burned!) on the bottom. Gently loosen the potstickers with a spatula, remove carefully, and place the potstickers *browned side up* on a platter or on individual dishes. Serve hot, with a selection of dipping sauces.

4 POTSTICKERS   EXCHANGES PER SERVING: 2 medium-fat meat; 1 starch; 1 vegetable   CALORIES: 260   PROTEIN: 16 gm   CARBOHYDRATE: 26 gm FAT: 9 gm   FIBER: 1.6 gm   CHOLESTEROL: 33 mg   SODIUM: 120 mg

DIPPING SAUCES

Use a selection of these sauces with both *siu mai* and potstickers.

MUSTARD. This is June's favorite. We've tried various brands of Chinese mustard, both prepared and dry, but the best we've come up with is Coleman's dry mustard mixed with milk. Even when you use nonfat, as we always do, it makes for a very creamy (and hot!) product, and it's diabetically free. Be careful not to add too much milk or it becomes so thin that it runs into the other sauces on your plate.

CHINESE RICE-WINE VINEGAR. This is another freebie, but be sure to use the mild variety.

CHILE OIL. Barbara's favorite. Available in major supermarkets or Asian specialty markets. Also diabetically free, especially since you don't dare use more than a few drops.

SOY SAUCE (if you can take the extra sodium). Use it either straight or with minced ginger or garlic.

PLUM SAUCE AND/OR HOISIN SAUCE. These are full of sugar and are to be used only to indulge the civilians in your dining group.

DR. BROWN'S CHINESE CHICKEN SALAD

SERVES 4

Chinese chicken salad is a popular favorite on Southern California menus. This version, by our friend Dr. Ron Brown, is particularly good and particularly healthy.

2 cups shredded cooked chicken
  ½ cup raw carrots
½ cup Chinese pea pods or
  sugar snap peas
  8 ounces sliced water chestnuts
  (canned)
½ bunch cilantro (optional)
1 cup raw bean sprouts
3 green onions, chopped
5 cups shredded lettuce
1 tablespoon toasted sesame seeds
2 tablespoons chopped walnuts

DRESSING:
3 tablespoons rice wine vinegar
2 tablespoons sesame oil (dark,
  if possible)
2 or 3 drops Tabasco sauce
½ teaspoon salt (optional)
Ground pepper to taste
½ packet Equal

Make the dressing by combining the rice vinegar (or white-wine vinegar), sesame oil, a few drops Tabasco, salt (optional), ground pepper to taste, and ½ packet Equal.

Mix half the dressing in a large bowl with the cooked chicken. Let marinate while you prepare the vegetables: toss together the carrots (cut into matchstick size), pea pods, water chestnuts, cilantro (optional), bean sprouts, green onions, and lettuce (the greener, the more nutritious). Toss with the chicken and the remainder of the dressing. Mix in sesame seeds and walnuts.

4 SERVINGS   EXCHANGES PER SERVING: 2 lean meat; 2 fat; 3 vegetable
CALORIES: 338   PROTEIN: 29 gm   CARBOHYDRATE: 19 GM   FAT: 17 gm
FIBER: 5 gm   CHOLESTEROL: 75 mg   SODIUM: 357 mg

WOKING YOUR WAY TO HEALTH. Wok cooking or stir-frying is healthy because you cook in such a very small amount of oil. And since you cook so fast and since most of the water or stock you cook in is evaporated or incorporated into the sauce, the vitamins and minerals are retained. It's also healthy because it takes so little time to do (once you've prepared the ingredients) that when you're in a hurry you're more likely to cook up something for yourself than resort to fast food or commercial frozen dinners.

For the best wok, buy a cheap steel one at least 12 inches in diameter. These are available in Asian markets. Don't buy a fancy electric one, because they heat up slowly and cannot be turned down quickly. If you don't already have a lid big enough to cover the wok, buy one. You'll also need a long-handled, scooplike stirrer with the bottom curved to match the shape of the wok. This is the standard wok tool used to shovel ingredients up and away from the hot spot in the bottom.

To cure your cheapie wok, if it has the usual lacquer coating, fill it with water, add 1 tablespoon baking soda, and boil for 15 to 20 minutes. Then it's easy to remove the coating with a plastic scouring pad. Dry the wok over low heat, and while it's hot, rub it with a paper towel moistened with vegetable oil.

After you use the wok, always soak it in hot water with detergent, scrub with a sponge or kitchen brush (never steel wool!), rinse, gently heat dry, and rub down with an oiled paper towel.

Over the months as you use your wok, it will start to turn black. Do not fret and do not clean the black off. For a wok, black is beautiful. It means it's well cured and better to cook in.

Although stir-frying comes to us from China, it can be used for any kind of cuisine. An excellent introductory book, *The Sunset Stir-Fry Cookbook,* has such non-Chinese recipes as Huevos Revueltos Rancheros, Pork Tenderloin Normandy, and Italian Stir-Fried Pasta.

STIR-FRYING VEGETABLES

To stir-fry fresh vegetables, simply prepare them by cutting them into small, uniform pieces or slices (so they cook fast and are all done at the same time). Then place the wok over high heat and add (for 2 cups of vegetables) ½ tablespoon of oil (preferably canola, avocado, or peanut). When the oil is hot put in all of the vegetables at once and stir for all you're worth for 1 minute. Add two tablespoons of water or chicken stock or beef broth. Slap on the lid and cook for about 3 to 5 minutes; we can't tell you exactly how long to cook because some kinds of vegetables cook faster than others and we don't know how well cooked you like your vegetables. Some trendy restaurants in Los Angeles serve their vegetables so raw they seem to be only barely heated. (These are the same ones that prefer fish to have a cool uncooked center because they have a deathly fear of drying it out.) You'll need to experiment to see what you and yours prefer. You can combine vegetables by either putting the ones that take less cooking time in later or by cooking them separately and then combining them at the end for a quick hot-hit.

If you double the amount of vegetables, double the amount of oil and liquid, but keep the cooking time the same.

To give your vegetables a Chinese taste, stir minced garlic and/or minced ginger into the oil before you add the vegetables, and add low-sodium soy sauce for half the liquid. To make the thicker sauce that you find in Chinese restaurants, instead of adding soy sauce and liquid and covering, make a mixture of ½ tablespoon cornstarch, ½ tablespoon water, ½ tablespoon low-sodium soy sauce, and ½ cup chicken broth. After stir-frying the vegetables, add this mixture and keep stirring until the sauce boils and becomes thick. But be careful not to cook it until it's dry and pasty.

CRAB IN BLACK-BEAN SAUCE

SERVES 4

When crab is on sale we usually make this dish. We particularly love it because you get down and dirty, eating with both your hands and licking your fingers. Also, since you're cracking the shells and picking out every last morsel of the sweet meat, you eat slowly, taking lots of time, and you have great feelings of satisfaction, although you're not eating all that much. (That's why we think eating artichokes is good for diabetics!)

*1 2-pound crab (or
  2 one-pound ones)
1½ tablespoons canned salted
  black beans
1 large or 2 small cloves garlic
1 teaspoon minced fresh
  ginger
¼ pound lean pork
  (optional)*

FOR THE SAUCE:
*1 tablespoon cornstarch
1 tablespoon low-sodium
  soy sauce
1 tablespoon dry sherry
½ cup chicken stock
1 egg, lightly beaten
3 green onions, chopped*

TO COOK:
3 tablespoons oil

PREPARING THE CRAB. The best way to prepare the crab is to have the butcher or fish-counter person clean and crack your crab for you. If he or she lacks the skill or time, you can do it yourself. (It's always good to learn a new kitchen skill, and once you've learned this one, besides making this more complex dish you can have a lovely simple meal of cracked crab served with lemon wedges, low-fat mayonnaise, and horseradish. But skip the cocktail sauce since that usually has sugar in it.)

Take the cooked crab and remove the top shell by grasping it and prying it off—it's not that difficult to do. You will see the gills, a kind of fingery fibrous material. Remove these with a sharp knife. Wash out all the rest of the stuff inside that can be washed out. Break off the claws and crack them with a hammer or mallet. Cut the body down the middle and then cut each half into three pieces, leaving the legs attached.

Rinse and drain the black beans (available in the Oriental-foods section of markets). Mash the beans and combine with the garlic (finely minced or put through a press) and ginger. To this mixture add the pork. (The pork is optional but gives a little extra protein, which may be needed in the diabetic diet.)

Prepare a sauce using the cornstarch, soy sauce, dry sherry (or Chinese wine, and lots of luck in finding it), and chicken stock. In another bowl combine the egg with the green onions.

Heat the wok and, when it is hot, add 3 tablespoons oil (peanut oil gives a distinctive Oriental taste, but avocado or canola are okay, too). When the oil is hot, add the pork and garlic-ginger mixture. Stir-fry briskly for about 2 minutes. Add the crab and stir-fry for another couple of minutes.

Add the cornstarch/soy/wine/chicken-stock sauce and keep stirring until the sauce boils and starts to thicken. Add the egg and green onions and stir-fry for about half a minute, or until the egg just starts to set. Serve instantly (have the guests waiting), with rice (white or brown as you prefer).

4 SERVINGS   EXCHANGES PER SERVING: 4 medium-fat meat; ½ starch;
CALORIES: 287   PROTEIN: 26 gm   CARBOHYDRATE: 9 gm   FAT: 15 gm
FIBER: 1.4 gm   CHOLESTEROL: 159 mg   SODIUM: 454 mg

Now we'll change directions and head east to the West, first touching down for some samples of our original favorite cuisine and one we still love, although in a different way than before.

FRANCE

French cooking has been somewhat out of favor in this country for a few years. People no longer want the rich sauces that it was famous for, and the lighter *cuisine minceur* never really caught on. But something good is happening to French cooking. French bistros are starting to pop up, and people (including us) really like the simpler peasant fare—and the lower prices. Here are a few favorite bistro-style recipes.

CÉLERI RÉMOULADE

SERVES 4

This is a classic and very satisfying French vegetable hors d'oeuvre that we've seldom seen in a restaurant or deli here. You can either go to France for it (try it at Scossa on the Place Victor Hugo in Paris) or make it yourself (it's no trouble). The only little obstacle is that its basic ingredient, celery root (celeriac), is usually available only in large markets, and it does take a food shredder or processor that can cut it into strips about one-eighth-inch wide.

1 large celery root

FOR THE DRESSING:
½ teaspoon Dijon mustard
2 tablespoons wine vinegar
⅓ cup salad oil

OR:
⅓ cup low-fat mayonnaise
½ teaspoon Dijon mustard

SERVE WITH:
Fresh chopped parsley

Pare off the fibrous outside of the celery root. Wash off any remaining dirt, and then cut it into chunks and shred it. Take your choice of dressings: (1) Dijon mustard beaten together with wine vinegar and salad oil; or (2) mayonnaise mixed with Dijon mustard. Mix the shredded celery root with as much of the dressing as your diet allows and chill. Serve with fresh chopped parsley sprinkled over the top. This makes a nice first course to serve with one of the following main courses.

4 SERVINGS   EXCHANGES PER SERVING: 2 fat; 1 vegetable   CALORIES: 106
PROTEIN: 5 gm   CARBOHYDRATE: 3 gm   FAT: 10 gm   FIBER: 1 gm
CHOLESTEROL: 0 mg   SODIUM: 60 mg

RAGOÛT D'AGNEAU À LA FRANÇAISE (AKA LAMB STEW)

SERVES 6

It must be true that simple pleasures are the best, for we've found that guests slosh compliments all over the table when we serve this simple lamb stew.

3 tablespoons olive or salad oil
2 pounds lean lamb
1 chopped onion
1 clove garlic
1 tablespoon flour
1½ cups chicken broth
1 crushed bay leaf
1 pinch marjoram
½ cup dry white wine

Salt and pepper to taste
8 small white onions, peeled
3 sliced carrots
3 medium potatoes, peeled and
  cut into chunks

SERVE WITH:
Fresh chopped parsley
French bread

Heat the oil in a large pot. Add the lamb cut into one-inch cubes. Often it's best to take the easy way out and use leg of lamb. Brown the lamb over a brisk flame; then take it out of the pan and set it aside. In about 1 tablespoon oil that you've left in the pot, sauté the onion and garlic (that you've put through a garlic press) until transparent and gold. Put the lamb back into the pot and sprinkle the flour over all. Pour in the chicken broth, add the bay leaf, a fat pinch of marjoram, the white wine, and salt and pepper to taste. Stir everything well, put the lid on the pot, and simmer for 30 to 35 minutes. Every once in a while skim off with a tablespoon any fat that may have accumulated on top.

At the end of this first cooking period, add the onions and let the pot continue to bubble lightly for another quarter of an hour. Throw in the carrots and potatoes. Continue cooking at the same slow rate for about another half hour, or until the vegetables are tender but not mushy. When you serve the stew, dust each portion generously with chopped fresh parsley.

Serve the stew with French bread with which to sop up the lovely juices. (To heat French bread, wet your hands, then dry them on your uncut loaf of bread and put it in a hot oven until the crust is crisp.)

6 SERVINGS   EXCHANGES PER SERVING: 4 medium-fat meat; 1½ fat; 1 starch; 1 vegetable   CALORIES: 496   PROTEIN: 47 gm
CARBOHYDRATE: 28 gm   FAT: 19 gm   FIBER: 4 gm   CHOLESTEROL: 135 mg
SODIUM: 318 mg

You don't need much else with this stew. Start the meal with a salad or the céleri rémoulade and end it with fruit.

ROAST CHICKEN

SERVES 6

This is the classic French bistro dish—with a difference. Select a nice plump roasting chicken. A free-range chicken is the best if you can find it, but if not, try to get a chicken that has at least been grown in your state or very close by. Avoid chickens that have been shipped from Alabama or Arkansas (unless you live in Alabama or Arkansas) and possibly have been sitting for a few days on a railroad siding.

5 large cloves garlic, minced
½ cup minced parsley
½ cup fresh herbs (thyme, basil,
   marjoram, oregano, and so
   on) or ¼ cup dried herbs
1 roasting chicken, about
   4 pounds

Vegetable oil
1 lemon

FOR BASTING:
Dry white wine or dry vermouth

Mince the garlic and combine with the parsley and the fresh herbs (thyme, basil, marjoram, oregano, and so on) or the dried herbs. Sometimes you can find mixtures of Provençal herbs in gourmet shops, and those work very well. Once we gave the recipe an Italian touch by stuffing the chicken with a combination of minced garlic, chopped fresh basil, and chopped pine nuts.

Preheat the oven to 450 degrees. Take the whole chicken in your bare hands and stuff the garlic mixture under the skin wherever you can. Stuff down from the neck and up from the nether regions—going clear up into the skin under the thighs and legs. (Yes, it *can* be done!) Wipe your hands on the chicken: you don't want to waste any of that lovely garlic mixture. Give the chicken a light vegetable-oil rubdown. Put the whole lemon into the cavity. Put the chicken into a roasting pan.

Turn the oven temperature down to 350 degrees, put the chicken in, and cook it about 20 minutes per pound. Baste it every 15 or 20 minutes with dry white wine or vermouth. It's done when the juices run clear when you stick a fork into what June calls "the hip." You'll find you've never had a more succulent, flavorful chicken, and the garlic turns quite sweet-tasting in the cooking.

6 SERVINGS   EXCHANGES PER SERVING: 5½ lean meat   CALORIES: 309
PROTEIN: 44 gm   CARBOHYDRATE: 5 gm   FAT: II gm   FIBER: I.3 gm
CHOLESTEROL: I34 mg   SODIUM: I35 mg

Another way to roast chicken for lovers of the "stinking rose" is to put 40 cloves of garlic (sometimes we've cheated and used only 25) into the cavity and roast it as above. The sweet garlic can be spread on French bread for a special treat, or you can slice it onto whatever vegetable you're serving (broccoli is particularly good) or chop it into mashed potatoes.

Once Barbara was asked what she thought of roasting a chicken with both the minced garlic under the skin and the 40 cloves in the cavity. She said she thought that would be perfect for a Halloween dinner since it would drive away any vampires that might be cruising the neighborhood.

POTATOES WITH A HEMINGWAY HEART

SERVES 6

The classic French accompaniment for the classic French roast chicken would be French-fried potatoes. In a fat-conscious world, however, deep-frying is out. We've tried lower-fat oven-fried compromises and found that they just didn't do the job—especially one that involved dipping the potatoes in beaten egg whites.

The better way to go, we think, is to try something different, something that also adds another classic French touch—leeks. (Many moons ago, we heard Dorothy Parker speak at a library conference, where she told the audience that during one period when Hemingway was living in France, he lived for six months on nothing but leeks. She then peered over her spectacles at the audience and added, "That's spelled l-e-e-k-s.") Since occasionally Hemingway might have been able to also afford a couple of potatoes, we've called this dish Potatoes with a Hemingway Heart.

1 pound leeks	*¼ cup chicken stock*
3½ tablespoons plus 2 teaspoons	*⅓ cup milk*
vegetable oil in all	*2 russet potatoes*

Split the leeks lengthwise and wash thoroughly to get any dirt or grit out. Slice the white part and about an inch of the green crossways into very thin slices. (You can do this by hand or in a food processor.) Heat 1½ tablespoons of the vegetable oil in a saucepan over medium heat, add the leeks, and sauté, stirring constantly, for 2 to 3 minutes (don't let them brown). Add the chicken stock, cover, and cook for 15 to 20 minutes, or until tender. (Check occasionally to make sure the leeks aren't getting dry.) Add the milk and cook, uncovered, until the liquid is reduced and thickened. Let cool. (The dish can be prepared in advance up to this point and kept cool in the refrigerator.)

Peel the potatoes and shred by hand or with the medium shredding disk of the food processor. Immediately plunge the potatoes into enough ice water to cover for 15 minutes. Drain thoroughly in a strainer or sieve and put the potatoes in the center of a dish towel. Roll up and twist the towel, wringing out every bit of water you can.

In a large, nonstick skillet with a tight-fitting lid, heat 2 tablespoons of the vegetable oil over a medium flame. Spread half the potatoes evenly over the bottom of the skillet, smoothing and pressing them gently with the back of a spoon. Spread the leek mixture evenly over the potatoes up to ½ inch of the edge. Spread the rest of the potatoes over the top, trying not to let any leeks show through. Press down gently, making a round cake about 10 inches in diameter. Cover and cook over medium heat. (Shake the pan occasionally to make sure the potatoes are not sticking). After about 5 minutes, take off the lid to let out the steam. Dry the inside of the lid with a towel. Cover and cook (shaking occasionally) another 5 minutes. Take off the lid (again wipe it dry) and check to see if the potatoes are golden brown on the bottom. If they aren't, cook a little longer.

Now here comes the tricky part, though it's not as tricky as it sounds. Put the lid on the pan and turn the pan upside down, letting the cake drop into the lid. If the pan is totally dry, put in the remaining 2 teaspoons of oil and stir it around until the surface is lightly coated. Slide the potato cake off the lid into the pan. (The brown crispy bottom is now on top.) Cook uncovered over medium-low heat until the new bottom is golden brown. Sprinkle with parsley and, since it's so pretty, serve it on a platter, cutting individual portions at the table.

This is a remarkably versatile dish. Once we didn't have any leeks so we used braised fennel. It was equally good. It would work with braised onions as well. If you have nothing to put in the middle, then put nothing in the middle and you'll have the famous Swiss potato dish Rösti.

Now we need a vegetable dish for our bistro meal—an easy one that can be made ahead of time. We need something like . . .

6 SERVINGS   EXCHANGES PER SERVING: 1 starch; 1 fat; 1 vegetable
CALORIES: 182   PROTEIN: 2.5 gm   CARBOHYDRATE: 23 gm   FAT: 10 gm
FIBER: 3 gm   CHOLESTEROL: 0 mg   SODIUM: 56 mg

MARTHA'S RATATOUILLE

SERVES 6

Martha Kuljian, a librarian friend of ours, once served us this vegetable dish of southern France. We instantly requested the recipe and have been making it ever since; you will, too, once you've tasted it.

2 tablespoons olive oil	*1 bell pepper*
1 tablespoon salt (optional)	*2 onions*
1 garlic clove, crushed	*2 teaspoons capers*
1 medium eggplant	*1 large can Italian plum tomatoes*
4 medium zucchini	*Parsley*

In Martha's very own words: "I use a 9-by-12-inch baking pan and line it with foil. Put the olive oil, salt (feel free to use 1 teaspoon or none), and crushed garlic in the bottom. Cut the eggplant into large pieces (2 inches or so) and toss in the oil. Cut the zucchini into ¼-inch slices, the pepper into large pieces, and the onions into eighths, I guess—anyway, into recognizable pieces. Add to the pan along with the capers (I buy mine from an Italian deli in bulk), and on top put the tomatoes. I don't use the juice at all; just cut each tomato into halves or quarters, depending on size. Fresh ones are great, too. Sprinkle with parsley, preferably fresh. Cover with foil and bake at 350 degrees for 1 hour or longer, until the onion is done. I always make this at least one day ahead. [Unlike Martha, we have been known to eat it right out of the oven.] It also is delicious cold or at room temperature, with a couple of teaspoons of balsamic vinegar added, and served on a lettuce leaf."

6 SERVINGS EXCHANGES PER SERVING: 1 fat; 1 vegetable   CALORIES: 80
PROTEIN: 2 gm   CARBOHYDRATE: 9 gm   FAT: 5 gm   FIBER: 3 gm
CHOLESTEROL: 0.8 mg   SODIUM: 1074 mg (with 1 tablespoon salt)

SHRIMP AU PERNOD

SERVES 4

This is a nice celebratory dish, because you can dazzle your guests—or yourself—by igniting the Pernod at the table. It's served at Los Angeles's historic Biltmore Hotel. Pernod, incidentally, is a yellow-colored, anise-flavored French aperitif. Barbara traditionally has a small glass of it her first night in Paris. (You fill the glass with water and the liquid becomes milky white.) You probably won't want to invest in a big bottle of Pernod. Just get one of those bottles like the ones they serve on airlines, and you'll have plenty to make the dish three or four times.

*2 tablespoons extra-virgin
  olive oil
3 to 4 tablespoons shallots,
  finely chopped
1 teaspoon chopped garlic
1 teaspoon chopped parsley*

*16 jumbo shrimp, peeled and
  deveined
2 tablespoons Pernod
Salt (optional), pepper,
  and cayenne*

Heat the olive oil in a skillet over medium heat. In the oil sauté the shallots, garlic, and parsley. To this add the shrimp and sauté until pink. Add the Pernod and ignite. (It lights more reliably if you warm it before adding.) Now season with a little salt (optional), pepper, and cayenne. *Voilà!* It's ready.

4 SERVINGS   EXCHANGES PER SERVING: 2 lean meat; 1½ fat
CALORIES: 133   PROTEIN: 6 gm   CARBOHYDRATE: 6 gm   FAT: 7 gm
FIBER: 0.1 gm   CHOLESTEROL: 43 mg   SODIUM: 44 mg

COUSCOUS

SERVES 4

Couscous is a good accompaniment for your shrimp dish and many other dishes as well. This quick, easy-to-prepare, and versatile product comes to France—and to us—via Morocco. Since it's made of hard durum wheat (as the best pastas are), you might call it a kind of granular pasta. The raisins are optional if you don't have the Fruit Exchange available or prefer to save it for your dessert.

¼ cup raisins (optional)	2 teaspoons lemon juice
1 tablespoon butter, margarine,	¼ teaspoon ground cumin
or avocado oil	1 cup couscous
½ cup finely chopped onion	Salt to taste (optional)
1½ cups boiling water	

Cover the raisins with lukewarm water for 15 to 20 minutes; drain and reserve for later use. Melt the butter, margarine, or oil in a saucepan and add the onion. Cook, stirring, over low heat until the onion is limp but not brown. Add the boiling water, lemon juice, ground cumin, and raisins. Bring to a boil, remove from the heat, and add the couscous. Add salt to taste (optional). Immediately clap on the lid and let stand for 5 minutes. Uncover, fluff with a fork, and serve.

4 SERVINGS   EXCHANGES PER SERVING: 1 starch; ½ fat   CALORIES: 108
PROTEIN: 2 gm   CARBOHYDRATE: 19 gm   FAT: 3 gm   FIBER: 2 gm
CHOLESTEROL: 8 mg   SODIUM: 35 mg

ITALY

Ah, home again, in Italy. We have such an affinity for Italian food these days that we're beginning to feel that in some previous incarnation we must have dwelt along the Arno or beside Lake Como or in a town clinging to a cliff above the Mediterranean. And it seems that most Americans share our passion for Italian cuisine. In survey after survey, Italian restaurants lead the list as the favorite place to dine. And Italian cuisine is healthy, what with its use of the monounsaturate olive oil and its emphasis on vegetables and pasta (which, for some wonderful reason, doesn't raise a diabetic's blood sugar as much as corresponding amounts of other complex-carbohydrate dishes as long as you don't overcook it. Make it *al dente*).

Italian cooking is also easy to do. As Biba Caggiano, owner and chef of one of Sacramento's best restaurants and author of *Northern Italian Cooking,* says, "Italian food is simply outstanding and outstandingly simple."

Getting involved with Italian cooking means, when you come home after a hard day, never having to resort to fast foods or going out to a restaurant in desperation. With a freezer containing a few balls of pizza dough, a bag of ravioli, and some containers of homemade tomato sauce and a cupboard containing pastas of various kinds, a bag of Arborio rice, some dried mushrooms, and bottles of extra-virgin olive oil and balsamic vinegar, you always have the makings of a healthy, easy-to-prepare dinner that you and your family will relish.

PIZZA FROM HELL (IT'S HEAVENLY!)

MAKES 4 8″–9″ PIZZAS

You can say about pizza what was once said about another pervasive element in society—you guess which: when it's good it's terrific, and even when it's not too great, it's still pretty good. To our minds and taste buds, pizza moved into the realm of terrific in a dark, cavernous restaurant called Inferno ("hell") in Madonna di Campiglio, an isolated ski resort in Italy. There we first experienced pizza made in an appropriately "hot as hell" wood-fired brick oven. Contrary to the restaurant's name, its pizza was pure heaven. June found she could eat twice as many slices of these crisp, thin-crusted disks of delight without going over her carbohydrate allotment as she could the pizza we were accustomed to back home. The toppings were much more interesting and generally more healthy than the fat-laden cheese-and-sausage-and-pepperoni variety usually available to us.

Once we returned home we often longed for such pizza. Our dreams came true when Alice Waters, of Chez Panisse in Berkeley, opened a café upstairs from the restaurant and began serving amazing pizza. The next time we went to the Bay Area, we went to the Chez Panisse café and had what was like the Pizza from Hell in Madonna di Campiglio: the product of a wood-fired brick oven, with a light and crispy crust and interesting toppings.

Not long after that, Wolfgang Puck put Los Angeles on the pizza map with his place on the Sunset Strip, Spago, where Hollywood movers and shakers made reservations a month in advance to try—among other culinary wonders—his duck-sausage pizza and later on down the line his smoked-salmon pizza.

The reason we're carrying on at such great length about pizza is that we want to inspire you to do as we now do—make an ever-changing panoply of Pizzas from Hell in your own kitchen. You'll find that the pizza you make is a hundred times better than what you've tried in the pizza chains and a thousand times more appropriate to the diabetic diet. You'll thrill and delight your friends.

To make Pizza from Hell, you will need to get a few tools of the trade: a peel (the large wooden paddle used to put the pizza in the oven and take it out; available by mail order from Williams-Sonoma, phone 1-800-541-2233; or from Sassafras, 1-800-537-4941) and a pizza stone or tiles (stones are also available from Sassafras; Salday Products has tiles set in a metal frame; 1-800-536-4941).

FOR THE YEAST MIXTURE:

1 package dry yeast
¼ cup warm water
½ teaspoon honey or
  brown sugar

2 tablespoons olive oil
1 teaspoon honey or
  brown sugar
3 cups all-purpose flour

FOR THE DOUGH:

¾ cup water
1 teaspoon salt

TO COAT THE DOUGH:

1 or 2 teaspoons of olive oil

Once you're well equipped, first make your dough. Dissolve the package of dry yeast in the warm water to which you've added either the honey or brown sugar. Remain calm. This little bit of honey or brown sugar won't hurt you; it's just to get the yeast working. Let it roil around for about 10 minutes.

In another mixing bowl combine the water for the dough with the salt, olive oil, and honey or brown sugar. (Again don't worry; most of this dissipates in the cooking.)

Put the flour in the bowl of a food processor, which you've fitted with a metal blade. (If you don't own a food processor, you can do this in a mixing bowl, using a spoon.) With the processor running, pour the water-salt-honey-oil mixture in through the tube. When this is all mixed in, pour in the dissolved yeast. Keep the processor running until the dough forms a smooth ball. If it's sticky, put in a little more flour.

On a *very* lightly floured board (only enough flour to keep the dough from sticking) knead the dough until it is smooth and shiny and elastic. This will take around 10 minutes. Then put a teaspoon or two of olive oil into a large bowl. Roll the ball of dough around in the oil until all the surface is coated. (You don't want a crust to form on the dough.) Cover the bowl with a dish towel and let rest in a warm place until the dough rises to about double in size.

Form the dough into a cylinder and divide it into four equal parts. Form each part into a ball and put it in a sealable plastic bag. Put the bags of dough into the refrigerator, where it will keep for up to two days. (You can freeze any dough you don't want to use right away. The morning of the day you plan to use frozen dough, take it out of the freezer and put it in the refrigerator to defrost.)

About half an hour before you intend to form your pizzas, place your pizza stone or tile on the lowest shelf of your oven. Turn the oven on as high as it will go and let it heat up for the half hour.

Before you start forming your pizzas, you should have your peel ready and lightly dusted with flour or cornmeal. Take a ball of dough that you've brought to room temperature, and on a lightly floured board roll it out until it's around 6 inches in diameter. Then stretch it until its diameter increases to about 8 or 9 inches. You can do this in one of three ways. (We once sat at the counter of Postrio, Wolfgang Puck's San Francisco outpost, and watched the pizza makers in action.) If you're a beginner you can either (1) pinch and stretch your way around the pizza with thumbs and index fingers (thumbs on one side, index fingers on the other; the pizza also stretches itself a little as it hangs down) or (2) rest the pizza on your two doubled-up, fists and stretch it by moving your fists apart; keep working in a circular motion. Gravity helps the stretching in this method, too.

The pros put the dough on their doubled-up fists as in method 2 and then spin it into the air—the higher, the more pro—several times until it's the desired size. Barbara, who does the pizza making, is cautiously starting to work on this method. She's now up to tossing it a mighty 4 or 5 inches.

Incidentally, if your pizza turns out to be oval or lopsided, don't let it bother you. In Italy, they sometimes make it that shape deliberately. It's called Pizza Rustica.

Okay, now it's on the peel. You may want to pinch up the edges a bit so your toppings don't slide off when you shoot it into the oven. Put on the toppings you select, open the oven door, and, with a shove forward and jerk back of the peel, shoot the pizza onto the stone or tiles. This sounds hard to do in contemplation, but it's really quite easy in execution.

How long do you bake your pizza? That pretty much depends on how hot your oven gets. It can range from 10 to 15 minutes. The best thing to do is just watch it. When the crust is golden brown, it's done. Slide your peel under the pizza and put the pizza on a round tray for serving and cutting with your roller-bladed pizza-cutting wheel. Cut each pizza into four servings.

4 SLICES   EXCHANGES PER SERVING: 1 starch   CALORIES: 95
PROTEIN: 2 gm   CARBOHYDRATE: 17 gm   FAT: 2 gm   FIBER: 0.5 gm
CHOLESTEROL: 0 mg   SODIUM: 134 mg

(There is no way we can calculate exchanges and nutrition facts for whatever toppings you choose for your pizza; we trust you can estimate them yourselves.)

TOPPINGS. As we pointed out above, when it comes to toppings you can put on just about anything you want. There are only a couple of restrictions. You don't want anything too wet, such as tomatoes that haven't had the seeds and juice squeezed out, or you'll make your beautiful crisp pizza into a soggy mess. You also don't want to put anything on the pizza that can't be cooked in around 15 minutes unless you cook it—or partially cook it—ahead of time.

To give you guidelines in choosing toppings, the following are some pizzas we serve when we're having our "panoply of pizzas" for guests.

SALMON APPETIZER PIZZA

Legend has it that Wolfgang Puck invented his salmon pizza once when, having no bagels on hand and seeking to appease someone wanting lox and bagels, he made a pizza and put the lox and sour cream on that. In our variation we make mini-pizzas by dividing the ball of dough into six parts and rolling each out and stretching it until it's about 2 to 2½ inches in diameter. Brush with olive oil. Put on a little finely chopped green onion or thinly sliced red onion. If you use the standard orange-colored smoked salmon (lox), cook the pizzas before you put it on. For a special treat, order your smoked salmon from Taku Smokeries of Juneau, Alaska. Call 1-800-582-5122 or log on to www.takusmokeries.com.

When you take the pizzas out of the oven, garnish each with a dollop of low-fat sour cream with a little dill (preferably fresh) and a little ground pepper. If it's a really festive occasion, you can top it with a demitasse spoonful of caviar.

CARAMELIZED ONIONS, BLUE CHEESE, AND ROSEMARY PIZZA

This is a variation on an Alice Waters recipe. We use much less onion (for diabetic purposes), and we're more flexible with the cheese: she specifies Gorgonzola, but it can just as well be blue cheese or Roquefort.

1 fairly large onion	*2 ounces blue cheese*
1 teaspoon butter, margarine,	*Rosemary*
or avocado oil	*Ground black pepper*
1 teaspoon olive oil	*Pancetta (optional)*

Slice the onion in the thinnest possible slices. Heat the butter, margarine, or avocado oil and the olive oil in a nonstick pan over the lowest heat. Add the onion and cook slowly, again on the lowest setting, until the onion is golden brown. (This may take as long as an hour. Just be sure the onion doesn't burn.)

When you're ready to make your pizza, spread the onions on the dough, dot the surface with blue cheese, and sprinkle with rosemary—preferably fresh. We go easy on the rosemary because many people aren't crazy about it and it can easily overwhelm the dish. When done, add a few coarse grindings of pepper. (When we feel we can afford the extra fat—which is seldom—we sometimes add a little pancetta, which we have cooked to the point of extreme crispiness in paper towels in the microwave.) We usually serve this with a green salad or a roasted-pepper salad.

SUN-DRIED TOMATOES, GARLIC, BLACK OLIVES, AND CHEESE PIZZA

Sun-dried tomatoes are handy to have in the cupboard when tomatoes aren't at their best. They also deliver a good tomato flavor without excessive liquid. Reconstitute the tomatoes according to the directions on the package.

3 ounces low-fat mozzarella	*Sun-dried tomatoes*
or dry Sonoma Jack cheese	*5 or 10 black olives, Niçoise,*
Chopped garlic	*Italian, or Greek*

Grate the mozzarella or dry Sonoma Jack cheese (California Gold Monterey Dry Jack, called *incomparable* by the *New York Times,* is similar in sharpness to a good moderately aged Parmesan; available from Vella Cheese Company, Box 191, Sonoma, CA 95476–0191; phone 1-800-848-0505), and sprinkle half of it on the pizza. Then top with a little chopped garlic, thin slices of the sun-dried tomatoes, and 5 big or 10 tiny chopped black olives of the Niçoise, Italian, or Greek persuasion. (We use locally cured Niçoise ones that we get at the farmer's market.) Sprinkle with the rest of the cheese. Cook as usual, serve as usual, enjoy as usual.

As you can see, we make very light toppings. They're more subtle that way and you can use the pizza more like a bread course and serve it with a regular protein course. That way a diabetic can get enough protein. Of course, you can always put more protein on the pizza—such as sausage, ham, chicken, and so forth—and make it a main course. Aidel's Sausage Company of San Francisco makes an amazing variety of lower-fat sausages containing no MSG, binders, extenders, fillers, or preservatives except for the sodium nitrite required by law in smoked products. Call 415-285-6660 for their tempting catalog and recipes.

You can make a calzone by putting your topping on only one half of the pizza dough and up to 1 inch from the edge, folding the unfilled side over, and, using a little water, pressing the edges together to seal. This puffs up beautifully in the oven.

You can also make great sandwich buns by dividing the ball of dough into thirds and rolling each third into a circle about 4½ inches in diameter. These, too, will puff up in the oven.

PASTA PERFECT

Take a look at the "Pasta, Corn, Rice, Bread" section of the Glycemic Index and you'll see which has the lowest number: pasta. That gives us one more reason to love this versatile carbohydrate. Though we used to make fresh pasta, we find that now we're happy with any of the good imported Italian pastas (Agnesi, De Cecco, D'Aquino).

To cook pasta, always boil it in a large pot with preferably 12 cups of water, even though you're cooking just enough for one or two. A little olive oil helps keep things from sticking. Add 1 teaspoon of salt to the boiling water, unless you're sodium-restricted. You can used the instructions on the package as a guideline, but you must keep testing so you'll know the moment it's right. Fish out a strand, run it under cold water, and bite into it to see if it's *al dente*—tender but not mushily soft, firm but not with a hard, raw-tasting heart. (According to diabetes specialist Dr. Alan Marcus of South Orange County, California, "Overcooked pasta raises blood sugar because the boiling water changes the starch into sugar.") When it has reached this ephemeral state, remove it immediately, drain it, place it in a prewarmed bowl, and toss with the sauce, which you've had the foresight to make ahead of time. Get the pasta to the table as fast as you can and serve it in individual prewarmed bowls or plates. *One-half cup cooked pasta (1 ounce dry) is 1 Starch/Bread Exchange.*

The sauce on your pasta can be as simple as Olive Oil and Garlic Sauce, or Tomato Sauce, or it can be a more complex one such as Putanesca Sauce. Note: be sure not to drown the pasta in sauce; the sauce should just delicately coat the pasta the way salad dressing is supposed to just coat the greens.

OLIVE OIL AND GARLIC SAUCE

MAKES ½ CUP SAUCE

2 teaspoons minced garlic
½ cup extra-virgin olive oil

FOR SERVING:
1 or 2 tablespoons of minced parsley
Ground pepper

Sauté the minced garlic over low heat in the olive oil. Stirring it so it doesn't burn, cook the garlic until it becomes a rich, golden color. Toss this sauce with your *al dente* pasta, along with a tablespoon or two of minced parsley and a few grinds of pepper.

A ONE-TABLESPOON SERVING EXCHANGES PER SERVING: 3 fat
CALORIES: 159 PROTEIN: 0 gm CARBOHYDRATE: 0 gm FAT: 18 gm
FIBER: 0 gm CHOLESTEROL: 0 mg SODIUM: 0 mg

TOMATO SAUCE

4 cups chopped tomatoes   *1 finely chopped onion*
1 tablespoon olive oil

Put the tomatoes—preferably homegrown or farmers'-market purchased—in a large bowl and pour boiling water over them to cover.
After only a half minute, quickly take out the tomatoes with a slot-
ted spoon and put them in a bowl of ice water (have a few cubes
floating in the water). After another half minute remove from water
and drain. Peel off the skin, slice the tomatoes across the middle (at
the equator), and squeeze out the juice and seeds. Chop the tomatoes
and, if they're still very juicy, drain in a colander or sieve. If you use
canned tomatoes, get the Italian kind and drain off the liquid before
chopping.

For every 4 cups of chopped tomatoes, sauté 1 finely chopped
onion in 1 tablespoon olive oil, over low heat, covered, for around 10
minutes. Add the tomatoes and cook over higher heat, stirring constantly, for 5 to 10 minutes, or until most of the loose juice is gone.
Process in a food processor. Use what you need and freeze the rest (it
lasts 6 to 12 months).

½-CUP SERVING   EXCHANGES PER SERVING: 1 vegetable   CALORIES: 36
PROTEIN: 1 gm   CARBOHYDRATE: 5 gm   FAT: 2 gm   FIBER: 1 gm
CHOLESTEROL: 0 mg   SODIUM: 8 mg

You can make infinite variations on your tomato sauce by adding
such things as herbs (fresh and dried), a couple of tablespoons of
milk or cream, sautéed garlic, Parmesan cheese, and so forth. This
sauce can be used on pizza as well as pasta, and it can be used as the
base sauce even for non-Italian recipes.

PASTA PUTANESCA

SERVES 4

2 cloves thinly sliced garlic
1½ tablespoons olive oil
3 anchovy fillets, or a 3-inch
    strip of anchovy paste
1 cup homemade tomato sauce,
    or 1 cup chopped canned
    Italian plum tomatoes
2½ teaspoons capers, rinsed
    and drained
6 Italian or Greek black olives,
    pitted and chopped

1 teaspoon chopped fresh parsley,
    or ½ teaspoon dried
1 teaspoon chopped fresh basil,
    or ½ teaspoon dried
1 teaspoon chopped fresh oregano,
    or ½ teaspoon dried
Red pepper flakes to taste
8 ounces pasta

Sauté the garlic in olive oil until golden. Add the anchovy fillets that have been rinsed and mashed along with the homemade tomato sauce (or Italian plum tomatoes), capers, black olives (if you use the tiny French Niçoise olives, use 12), fresh parsley, basil, and oregano, and the red-pepper flakes to taste. Simmer gently 10 to 15 minutes. Cook the 8 ounces of pasta and toss with the sauce.

4 SERVINGS EXCHANGES PER SERVING: 2 starch; ½ medium-fat meat; 1 fat; 1 vegetable CALORIES: 287 PROTEIN: 9 gm CARBOHYDRATE: 48 gm FAT: 7 gm FIBER: 5 gm CHOLESTEROL: 0 mg SODIUM: 94 mg

Your pasta becomes a main course with all the protein you need when you make the following:

BOLOGNESE SAUCE

SERVES 4

2 tablespoons butter or
   margarine
2 tablespoons olive oil
½ cup finely chopped onion
2 tablespoons finely chopped
   carrot
2 tablespoons finely chopped
   celery
¾ pound ground lean beef
¾ pound ground turkey

1 cup dry white wine or white
   vermouth
½ cup nonfat milk
2 cups fresh tomatoes, or 2 cups
   chopped canned Italian
   plum tomatoes

SERVE WITH:
Grated Parmesan or Romano
   cheese

In a large, preferably enamel, pot or saucepan, heat the butter or margarine and olive oil. Add the onion, carrot, and celery. Sauté over medium heat until translucent and just barely starting to brown. Add the ground beef and ground turkey. Cook, stirring, until the meat loses its pink color. Add the white wine or white vermouth and cook over medium-high heat until the wine has evaporated. Add the milk and continue cooking until that has evaporated. Add the fresh tomatoes that have been peeled and seeded (see Tomato Sauce recipe) or canned tomatoes with their juice. Cover and, over low heat, simmer gently, stirring occasionally, for 2 hours, or until the sauce thickens. Rather than tossing the sauce with the pasta, put your pasta allotment in a heated bowl and top with your allotment of Bolognese Sauce. Sprinkle with grated Parmesan or Romano cheese.

½-CUP SERVING   EXCHANGES PER SERVING: 2 medium-fat meat; 1 fat; ½ vegetable   CALORIES: 192   PROTEIN: 14 gm   CARBOHYDRATE: 3 gm FAT: 13 gm   FIBER: 0.6 gm   CHOLESTEROL: 49 mg   SODIUM: 74 mg

RAVIOLI

An excellent way to create new and interesting dishes and even to use leftovers is to make ravioli. But we confess that until recently we found ravioli something of a chore to make, and they often turned out too thick and heavy. Finally, benevolent gods intervened and whispered, "Look on the Internet." There, under the heading, "wonton ravioli," we found numerous recipes. We use the round wonton wrappers, called zyoza, which are available at most large markets. Stuffed and sealed, these make perfect paper-thin ravioli.

We've been making and freezing quick and easy ravioli ever since. All you do is mix up your filling of choice and put the wonton skin in the middle of a dumpling/ravioli maker (the same one we recommended for making potstickers). Put 1 teaspoon of the filling in the middle of the wonton skin, brush the edges with beaten egg white, close the dumpling/ravioli maker firmly, open it, and there's your perfect ravioli (or would that be *raviolo?*). As you form your ravioli, keep them covered with a towel so they don't dry out. When you're ready, cook them in a large pot of gently boiling water, without crowding, for two minutes, or until they rise to the surface. As they are cooked, drain them on a paper towel and keep them warm until you have all you need for that meal. Freeze the rest of the uncooked ravioli. For the filling you may want to try some things like the following.

CHARD (OR SPINACH) AND CHEESE FILLING

SERVES 7

3 tablespoons finely chopped onion

2 tablespoons vegetable oil or margarine

2 cups chopped cooked spinach or chard

1 cup ricotta

1 beaten egg white

½ cup grated Parmesan, Romano, or dry Jack cheese

⅛ to ¼ teaspoon nutmeg

Sauté, until soft, the onion in vegetable oil or margarine. Add the spinach or chard, which you've squeezed all the moisture out of, and cook for 2 minutes. In a mixing bowl combine the spinach or chard mixture with the ricotta, beaten egg white, grated cheese, and nutmeg.

7 SERVINGS   EXCHANGES PER SERVING OF 4 ravioli: 1 starch; 1 medium-fat meat; 1 fat; ½ vegetable   CALORIES: 212   PROTEIN: 9 gm CARBOHYDRATE: 24 gm   FAT: 9 gm   FIBER: 1 gm   CHOLESTEROL: 16 mg SODIUM: 221 mg

MEAT FILLING

2 cups ground cooked beef, pork, chicken, or turkey
3 tablespoons finely chopped onion
1 clove finely chopped garlic
2 tablespoons olive or vegetable oil

2 tablespoons finely chopped parsley
1 beaten egg white
¼ cup grated cheese
Salt to taste (optional)
Freshly ground pepper to taste

Begin with 2 cups of any one or a combination ground cooked meat. (Use leftovers when you can.) Cook the onion and garlic in the olive or vegetable oil until the onion and garlic are soft but not brown. Add the ground meat and cook, stirring, for 1 minute. Remove from the heat and mix in the parsley, egg white, cheese, salt (optional), and freshly ground pepper to taste.

7 SERVINGS   EXCHANGES PER SERVING OF 4 ravioli: 1 starch; 2 medium-fat meat; 1 fat   CALORIES: 277   PROTEIN: 16 gm   CARBOHYDRATE: 21 gm FAT: 14 gm   FIBER: 0 gm   CHOLESTEROL: 109 mg   SODIUM: 51 mg

SWEET-POTATO FILLING

SERVES 6–7

1¾ pounds cooked sweet
   potatoes, pureed
½ cup grated cheese
3 tablespoons finely chopped
   parsley

2 tablespoons chopped ham,
   preferably prosciutto (optional)
2 beaten egg whites
¼ to ½ teaspoon nutmeg
Salt to taste (optional)

Combine the cooked sweet potatoes, which you have pureed in a
food processor until smooth, with the grated cheese, finely chopped
parsley, chopped ham, beaten egg whites, nutmeg, and salt to taste.
Mix thoroughly.

6 TO 7 SERVINGS   EXCHANGES PER SERVING OF 4 ravioli: 1 starch;
1 medium-fat meat   CALORIES: 239   PROTEIN: 7 gm
CARBOHYDRATE: 46 gm   FAT: 3 gm   FIBER: 2 gm   CHOLESTEROL: 7 mg
SODIUM: 264 mg

SAUCES FOR RAVIOLI

Use anything you like: just a little butter or margarine and grated
cheese, Tomato Sauce (with or without added herbs), Tomato Sauce
smoothed out with a little milk, Bolognese Sauce (don't use with
meat ravioli as that would be not only redundant but also boring),
pesto sauce (blend 1 cup fresh basil, ¼ cup olive oil, 1 tablespoon pine
nuts, 1 large clove garlic, and 3 to 4 tablespoons grated cheese), and
anything else your active imagination dictates.

RISOTTO. To our minds, risotto is the most wonderfully rich and
creamy of all the world's rice dishes. The most praised of all Italian
cookbook authors, Marcella Hazan, calls risotto "a uniquely Italian
technique for cooking rice . . . almost a cuisine all by itself." We can
only share with you here its most famous form, Risotto alla Milanese
(risotto in the Milan style) and one variation, plus a few ideas for

others. Risotto should be made with unwashed Arborio rice from northern Italy. (California's short-grained pearl rice is okay, too.)

The method for cooking risotto differs from all other rice-cooking methods in that the liquid is added a small amount at a time. It is truly a handcrafted dish in the sense that you stand and stir for at least 20 minutes until the rice becomes, in Hazan's words, "a creamy union of tender, yet firm grains." But we find that risotto can be made quickly, easily, and reliably in the microwave. The secret is to cook the rice for a total of only about 18 minutes, stirring only two or three times.

RISOTTO ALLA MILANESE

SERVES 4

1 small onion, minced
3 tablespoons butter or
   avocado oil
1 cup Arborio rice
1 cup chicken stock

1 cup dry white wine
Dash ground saffron

FOR SERVING:
⅓ cup finely grated Parmesan cheese
Salt and pepper to taste

Combine the onion with the butter (or avocado oil) in a 2½-quart microwave casserole dish. Cover with wax paper and microwave on high for about 3 minutes, or until the onion is translucent. Mix in the rice, cover with wax paper, and microwave on high for 1 minute. Mix together chicken stock, white wine, and a dash of ground saffron. Add to the rice, cover with a tight lid, and microwave on high for 5 to 7 minutes, or until boiling. Stir. Put the lid on and microwave on medium for 9 to 10 minutes, or until almost all the liquid is absorbed and the rice tastes *al dente* (firm to the bite). Cover again and let stand 5 minutes. Just before serving, take a fork and stir in Parmesan cheese; add salt and pepper to taste.

4 SERVINGS EXCHANGES PER SERVING: 2 starch; ½ medium-fat meat; 2 fat CALORIES: 290 PROTEIN: 7 gm CARBOHYDRATE: 39 gm FAT: 11 gm FIBER: 1 gm CHOLESTEROL: 30 mg SODIUM: 246 mg

WINDSOR'S WHITE-WINE RISOTTO

SERVES 6

We've tried several microwave recipes, but find that this one, courtesy of Windsor Vineyards of California, is the best. We particularly like it with peeled and seeded tomatoes we've just picked out of our own yard, instead of the canned ones.

½ cup olive oil
½ medium onion, chopped
2 cloves garlic, chopped
1½ cups Arborio rice
1½ cups chicken broth
½ cup white wine

Juice of half a lemon
1 8-ounce can Italian plum
   tomatoes, drained

TO SERVE:
½ cup grated Parmesan cheese

Heat the olive oil in a skillet and sauté the onion and garlic. Add the rice, stirring until the rice grains turn opaque. Mix the chicken broth with white wine and lemon juice in a measuring cup. Then pour the contents of the skillet into a large microwave casserole dish with a top, adding the tomatoes. Add one-third of the liquid mixture from the measuring cup. Put the top on the casserole dish and cook in the microwave at high for 5 minutes.

Remove the dish and stir gently so that no rice is sticking to the bottom. Then add another third of the liquid and cook on high for 5 more minutes. Remove from the microwave and stir, adding the rest of the liquid, and microwave for 5 more minutes. Remove and stir a third time. The rice should be creamy, with a small amount of liquid. Stir in Parmesan cheese and serve.

6 SERVINGS EXCHANGES PER SERVING: 2 starch; 3½ fat;
½ medium-fat meat; ½ vegetable CALORIES: 380 PROTEIN: 7 gm
CARBOHYDRATE: 40 gm FAT: 20 gm FIBER: 1 gm CHOLESTEROL: 6 mg
SODIUM: 220 mg

OTHER IDEAS

WITH FRESH MUSHROOMS. Sauté about 4 ounces of mushrooms in oil or butter. Proceed with the Risotto alla Milanese recipe, adding the mushrooms at the end, when you add the cheese.

WITH DRIED PORCINI MUSHROOMS. Soak ½ ounce porcini mushrooms in warm water for 20 minutes; drain, rinse, and squeeze. Reserve the liquid and substitute it for part of the chicken stock in either risotto recipe (a little goes a long way). Add the mushrooms as above.

Asparagus, peas, spinach, or zucchini can also be used. Usually the vegetables are cooked first and added at either the beginning or the end. For guidance it's best to consult a good Italian cookbook—our current favorite being *Northern Italian Cooking* by Biba Caggiano (HP Books). Biba is the owner and chef of an outstanding restaurant in Sacramento, the eponymous (we've always wanted to use that word!) Biba's. Under her gentle guidance, you may even want to venture making risotto the classic way. And you certainly should try her other wonderful recipes. We particularly recommend her stuffed chicken breasts (slightly modified for the diabetic diet).

STUFFED CHICKEN BREASTS BIBA

SERVES 6

3 whole chicken breasts
3 paper-thin slices prosciutto
3 thin slices fontina or 3 table-
  spoons Parmesan cheese
1½ sage leaves
Milk
Flour
3 tablespoons butter
  or margarine

1 tablespoon olive oil
1 crushed chicken bouillon
  cube
1 cup dry white wine in all
Salt (optional)
Freshly ground pepper
  to taste
⅓ cup whipping cream, whole
  milk, or nonfat milk

Skin, bone, and split the chicken breasts; pound them a bit to flatten. Put a slice of prosciutto; a slice of fontina or a tablespoon of Parmesan cheese; and half a sage leaf on each breast. Roll up the breasts and secure them with wooden toothpicks. Dip them in milk, then roll in flour to lightly coat. Melt the butter or margarine in the olive oil. When butter or margarine foams, add the chicken breasts. Cook over medium heat until golden on all sides. Add the crushed chicken bouillon cube and ½ cup of the white wine. Add salt (optional) and freshly ground pepper to taste. When wine is reduced by half, add the remaining white wine. Cover skillet and reduce heat. Simmer 15 to 20 minutes, or until chicken is tender. Turn chicken several times during cooking. Add a little more wine if the sauce looks too dry.

Place chicken on a warm platter. Increase heat and add the whipping cream, milk, or nonfat milk (depending on how many Fat Exchanges you can afford to use). Deglaze the skillet by stirring to dissolve meat juices attached to the bottom. Taste the sauce and adjust the seasoning; then spoon it over the chicken. Serve immediately.

6 SERVINGS   EXCHANGES PER SERVING: 2 medium-fat meat; 2 fat
CALORIES: 271   PROTEIN: 28 gm   CARBOHYDRATE: 0.5 gm   FAT: 15 gm
FIBER: 0 gm   CHOLESTEROL: 102 mg   SODIUM: 198 mg

Finishing our Italian adventure on this culinary high point, we wish you *buon apetito e buona vita!*

· Desserts—Sweet Somethings ·

Desserts are notorious comfort foods. (That's what gets people into so much trouble with them!) Although we usually find our food comforts elsewhere, we always serve them to guests. And June usually plays dessert chef since in that way she has total control over content and portion size. Here are desserts she particularly enjoys making— and eating—and so do our guests.

RICE PUDDING

SERVES 6

The Grill on the Alley, a posh Beverly Hills restaurant near Rodeo Drive, has created Southern California's most popular rice pudding, and we've finally perfected our own diabetic version of it. Barbara likes it for breakfast and June likes it for lunch or a snack, and everybody likes it for dinner dessert. To escalate this pudding into the realm of the exotic, use perfumy Indian basmati rice instead of ordinary white rice.

¼ cup raisins
1 tablespoon butter
3½ cups milk
½ cup white rice
1 ½-inch piece of vanilla bean
1 cinnamon stick

4 packets of a non-caloric
sweetener that remains stable
in heat (Splenda, Sweet One,
DiabetiSweet, or Sunette)
1 egg yolk
2 tablespoons water

First boil the raisins for 3 minutes in water to cover. Allow these to cool while you're doing the rest. In a one-gallon saucepan put the butter, milk, rice, piece of vanilla bean, cinnamon stick, and packets of Sweet One. Bring to a boil and simmer 8 minutes, stirring every 2 or 3 minutes. Then beat the egg yolk with 2 tablespoons water and stir this into the rice. Simmer 10 minutes longer, stirring occasionally. Remove the vanilla bean and cinnamon stick and put the pudding into a refrigerator container, add the drained raisins, and refrigerate for 2 to 3 hours. Serve in half-cup containers, garnished with cinnamon.

6 SERVINGS   EXCHANGES PER SERVING: ½ starch; ½ medium-fat meat; ⅓ fruit   CALORIES: 139   PROTEIN: 6 gm   CARBOHYDRATE: 21 gm   FAT: 3 gm   FIBER: 0.5 gm   CHOLESTEROL: 43 mg   SODIUM: 96 mg

NOT-SO-NAUGHTY MUD *CAKE*

SERVES 8

Those of you who've traveled to the island of Kauai may have seen a diabetically sinful dessert called Naughty Hula Pie on the menu at the Kiahuna Plantation restaurant. Our mud cake is not so naughty as that, but it is a close relative and to be used only as a rare treat. Its fat content is beyond redemption, so we don't even try to do a modified version except for using fructose instead of sugar.

We discovered this recipe through Ruth Reichl, food editor of the *Los Angeles Times,* who in turn got it from the *Fanny Farmer Baking Book.* Here's her description of it: "This cake is about as easy as a cake can be. You can mix the batter right in the pan that you melt the chocolate in, so there's no bowl to wash. The cake needs no frosting. Best of all, it tastes completely wonderful. It's dark and dense, with a sophisticated flavor that no mix ever had."

*4 one-ounce squares
    unsweetened chocolate
6 tablespoons butter
¾ cup strong-brewed coffee
2 tablespoons bourbon
2 eggs
½ teaspoon vanilla extract
1¼ cups cake flour*

*½ cup granular fructose
½ teaspoon baking soda
⅛ teaspoon salt*

SERVE WITH:
*Vanilla ice cream or
    unsweetened whipped cream*

Combine the unsweetened chocolate, butter, and coffee in a heavy saucepan. Heat over very low heat until the chocolate melts, stirring until smooth and blended. Cool 10 minutes. Beat in the bourbon, eggs, and vanilla extract.

Sift the cake flour with the fructose, baking soda, and salt. Add to chocolate mixture, beating until smooth. Pour into a greased and floured 8-by-4-inch loaf pan. Bake at 275 degrees for 45 to 55 minutes. Cool in the pan for 15 minutes, then turn out onto a rack and allow to cool completely.

Serve with a vanilla ice cream or a tiny bit of unsweetened whipped cream.

8 SERVINGS   EXCHANGES PER SERVING: 1 starch; 1½ fat; ⅓ milk
CALORIES: 202   PROTEIN: 4 gm   CARBOHYDRATE: 34 gm   FAT: 6 gm
FIBER: 1 gm   CHOLESTEROL: 103 mg   SODIUM: 103 mg

SWEET POTATOES DULLES

SERVES 6

Our name for this dessert comes from where we discovered it: the Hyatt Hotel at Dulles Airport, where we spent the night prior to taking an early-morning flight.

This unusual dessert actually wasn't planned as a dessert. It was a side dish served with one of the main courses. Since it was made with sweet potatoes, which occupy a place much lower on the Glycemic Index than you would expect considering their sweet taste, we wanted to try it, but it wasn't served as part of either main course we were ordering. The amiable waitress was kind enough to make a substitution for us so we could have a taste. With the first bite we realized that with minor adjustments it would make a fabulous dessert. The chef was kind enough to write up the recipe for us. We use Fruit Sweet instead of honey and condensed nonfat milk instead of cream, but we think it tastes just as great as the original.

1 cup cooked sweet potatoes
1 egg
2 egg whites
1 cup condensed nonfat milk
⅛ teaspoon salt
3 tablespoons Fruit Sweet*

1 teaspoon cinnamon (or to taste)

SERVE WITH:
*Yogurt or sugar-free whipped
    topping*

In a food processor, combine the sweet potatoes with the whole egg and egg whites and process until smooth. Place this puree in a bowl

*To find in your area or to order directly: Wax Orchards 1-800-634-6132; www.waxorchards.com; e-mail: customerservice@waxorchards.com.

and whisk in the condensed milk, salt, Fruit Sweet (available from Wax Orchards; call 1-800-634-6132), and cinnamon.

Preheat the oven to 325 degrees. Spray thoroughly 6 small ramekins or custard cups with Pam and fill ¾ full with the potato batter. Place the cups in an ovenproof pan and add hot water to the pan to a level halfway up the cups. Bake for 35 to 40 minutes, or until a knife inserted in the potatoes comes out clean.

Either serve in the cups or turn them upside down on a plate. (You may have to put the cups in hot water and/or run a knife blade around the outside edge to loosen the potatoes.) Sweet Potatoes Dulles is delicious by itself, or you can top it off with a little yogurt or sugar-free whipped topping.

6 SERVINGS   EXCHANGES PER SERVING: ½ starch; ½ milk   CALORIES: 105
PROTEIN: 6 gm   CARBOHYDRATE: 18 gm   FAT: 1 gm   FIBER: 1 gm
CHOLESTEROL: 37 mg   SODIUM: 154 mg

And now we need a little bistro dessert. We'll make it light, we'll make it . . .

PEARS AMANDINE

SERVES 6

1 cup water
2 or 3 drops vanilla extract or
    1 inch of vanilla bean
3 packets Sweet One

3 fresh, ripe, but firm pears
1 cup sliced strawberries
2 or 3 slivers of toasted almond

Boil the water to which you've added the vanilla extract or vanilla bean and the packets of Sweet One. In this mixture poach for 8 minutes the pears, halved and cored. Remove the pears and place, flat side down, on a plate to cool.

Reduce the poaching syrup by simmering down to about ½ cup. Add the strawberries and boil until you have a nice syrupy syrup.

Pour into the blender or food processor and whirl until smooth. Stick a few slivers of toasted almond into each pear half and spoon some strawberry sauce over it. Refrigerate until serving time.

6 SERVINGS   EXCHANGES PER SERVING: I fruit   CALORIES: 56
PROTEIN: 0.5 gm   CARBOHYDRATE: 14 gm   FAT: 0.5 gm   FIBER: 3 gm
CHOLESTEROL: 0 mg   SODIUM: I mg

If you want to step a bit off the fruit route, cover poached pears with Fudge Sweet (available from Wax Orchards; call 1-800-634-6132).

You and Your Doctor

Although we've repeatedly pointed out that your diabetes control and your total health are primarily your responsibility, you can't do it alone. For the best therapy you need the help of a whole team of dedicated diabetes health professionals, and your co-captain of that team is your physician. Since diabetics work more closely (and longer!) with their doctors, they need to be particularly certain that they have just the right one.

If you have any doubts about the kind of care you're getting from your doctor, you might look over these twelve warning signs. They're from the book *Playing God: The New World of Medical Choices* by Drs. Thomas Scully and Celia Scully. They seem to us to be especially significant for diabetics.

CLUES YOU'RE NOT GETTING THE CARE YOU SHOULD*

Your doctor:

1. Doesn't seem to be listening to what you are telling him or her.
2. Doesn't answer your questions or take time to ask if you have any. When an answer is given, it is in words you don't understand.
3. Fails to take an adequate medical history or give you a complete physical examination when it is called for.
4. Doesn't help you learn more about your condition and what you can do about it, and gives no explanation as to why the recommended tests, treatment, or medications might be necessary.

*Reprinted from *Playing God: The New World of Medical Choices* by Thomas Scully and Celia Scully (New York: Simon and Schuster, 1987, pp. 43–44).

5. Neglects to inform you of potential risks, benefits, and side effects of prescribed drugs or suggested procedures and tests. (Beware if you have told your physician that you are allergic to a certain medication and it is prescribed anyway.)

6. (*for women*) Doesn't respect your modesty and makes suggestive remarks while doing a pelvic examination or examining your breasts.

7. Fails to make a follow-up appointment for you and does not instruct you to call the office to report on how you are doing.

8. Seems forgetful, peculiar, or belligerent, or has alcohol on his or her breath.

9. Is hard to reach, doesn't return phone calls, and fails to arrange for another doctor to care for you when he or she is out of town.

10. Is not on the staff of any community hospital or medical center.

11. Is rigid, acts as if he or she knows it all, and insists that the only way to treat your condition is his or her way.

12. Reacts defensively when you suggest a second opinion.

Another warning signal we might add is if your doctor doesn't practice *preventive* medicine.

The *First Surgeon General's Report on Health Promotion and Disease Prevention* declares that "prevention is a health idea whose time has come." We echo that declaration and, strangely enough, while we were formulating our own ideas on preventing diabetes problems through a total-health program, June received this letter from her doctor.

Dear Patients:

We would like to tell you of a shift in the emphasis in our practice. This change will be gradual and will not jeopardize our individual relationships with our patients, but should enhance the existing personalized treatment.

For many years our primary interest in medicine has been the prevention and treatment of cardiovascular disease and diabetes, particularly coronary disease, high blood pressure, heart attack, and stroke. Clinical research now available, in combination with our experience of the last thirty years, has produced convincing evidence that it is possible to detect and recognize certain Risk Factors which are often associated with these diseases. Fortunately, many of these Risk Factors can be altered favorably by the proper use of diet, medication, and healthful changes in habits and lifestyle. Proper control of these Risk Factors may prevent, defer, or ameliorate these diseases.

The most important Risk Factors which *can* be influenced favorably are *high blood pressure, cigarette smoking, high blood fats* (cholesterol, triglycerides, lipoproteins), and *diabetes.* Other Risk Factors which can be treated are *obesity, excessive stress,* and *lack of proper exercise.*

Risk Factor Reduction offers the greatest promise in the prevention of cardiovascular disease and diabetes. Our practice in the future will stress preventive medicine through Risk Factor Detection and Reduction in an integrated program for all our patients.

In the field of diagnosis, more time will be spent on very detailed history-taking and physical examination. Laboratory studies will include, in addition to the usual studies, treadmill stress tests, blood-lipid studies, and appropriate cardiac monitoring. Further diagnostic tests will be done where indicated.

After completion of these studies, a personal conference will be arranged to discuss, in detail, results and diagnoses and to give careful instructions concerning medications, diet, exercise, and other aspects of lifestyle. With our active cooperation and participation, patients will be deeply involved in assuming more responsibility for their own health. Periodic checkups will be performed to evaluate individual progress.

The prevention and treatment of cardiovascular disease and diabetes are most effective if begun early in one's life. Therefore new patients entering our practice will generally be under the age of fifty.

Patients of all ages who are already in our practice have our assurance that we will continue to care for them as in the past with even greater attention to our philosophy of Risk Factor Detection and Reduction. As always, if an emergency medical problem should arise, our office will be available for appropriate care and advice.

We will be of greater service to our patients by this expanded approach in our practice of Cardiology and Internal Medicine.

If you have any questions or comments we would like very much to hear from you.

We believe that by using this book and working closely with your own doctor and other diabetes health-care professionals you can create your own health-enhancement program and do it in the area in which you're going to be practicing it—your own environment and your own daily life.

A survey by Louis Harris showed that a majority of Americans would like their doctors to advise them on preventive health measures but that only a small minority of doctors do so. We don't blame the doctors for this. We say, along with the warden in the film *Cool Hand Luke,* "What we have here is a failure to communicate." Probably that majority of Americans never *tell* the doctor they'd like advice on preventive health measures. We think that if you do tell your doctor you'll get nothing but enthusiastic cooperation. (You might even show him or her June's doctor's letter.)

As part of your prevention program with your doctor we think you should have an understanding program. That is to say, we think you should ask for a full explanation of all test results. For example, you shouldn't just know that your blood sugar is "okay" or your cholesterol is "average for your age" or your triglycerides are "a little on the high side." You should know the exact numbers and understand their significance. (This also gives you a basis for comparison for the future improvement you're bound to have with your new lifestyle.) In explaining these figures and other aspects of your health to you, your doctor needs to become as much a teacher as a healer. Barbara Brown, the biofeedback expert, warns that this is the hardest shift for some doctors to make, because it is a new role for them. But we feel that when they do learn to share their knowledge and the responsibility for your good health with you, both of you will gain.

We also think you should ask your doctor to recommend a dietitian if there isn't one on staff. You should work with this dietitian on planning your individual diet, especially if you intend to make any deviations from the standard Exchange Lists. In our opinion, a dietitian is one of the most vital (and unfortunately one of the most frequently missing) members of your total-health-program team. Most doctors have neither the time, the inclination, nor the background to give you the individual dietary counseling you need to bring about optimum health and control.

If your doctor doesn't have the name of a dietitian for you, call your local hospital and ask the dietitian there for a referral, or contact the American Dietetic Association, 120 South Riverside Plaza, Suite 2000, Chicago, IL 60606-6995, 312-899-0040 or http://eatright.org/finddiet.html. You can also reach a dietitian specializing in diabetes through the American Association of Diabetes Educators, 100 West Monroe Street, Suite 400, Chicago, IL 60603, 800-338-3633 or www.aadenet.org. Click on "Find an Educator," then click on your state and go to your city. Look for those who have R.D., CDE after their name.

Another thing we heartily recommend is taking a diabetes-education course. Most of these are reasonably priced and some are even free. At these courses you receive instruction from doctors, nurses, and dietitians and sometimes from social workers, psychologists, and exercise therapists. Call your local diabetes association to find out what courses are available in your area or write or call the American Association of Diabetes Educators, 444 North Michigan Avenue, Suite 1240, Chicago, IL 60611; phone 1-800-338-DMED.

Get busy working out your prevention program. Do it now! The life you enhance and prolong will definitely be your own.

Index